Creativity in Nursing

(and Other Professions)

Shirley M. Steele, R.N., Ph.D.
University of Texas School of Nursing
Galveston, Texas
and
Frank L. Maraviglia, M.S.
State University of New York
Environmental Science and Forestry
School of Landscape Architecture
Syracuse, New York

26285

The Art of Being Human

What is all this current clamor:
Be more human in our manner
In caring for the sick, the well—
Have we not done so for a spell?

We've expanded science and technology
Found new secrets in biology.
The heart of science: our concern
The art of being human: later learn.

Science helps the sick recover
Secrets of a longer life: discover!
But when the end for each arrives
Science succumbs-art survives.

How we live, how healthy we become
Is more art than science for some
The science of wellness-less well known
Than the science of sickness with which we've grown.

As health professionals we've much to learn
About health care as a joint concern.
Is it science or art that is most potent?
An endless debate with no rapprochement.

Some special knowledge need I learn
To specialize in this new concern?
Personal growth and awareness required
To become the person you once aspired.

To laugh, to cry, to touch, to feel
Has little scientific appeal.
The art of being human needs reflection
As you prepare to enter your profession.

A creed to guide your future direction
Nursing requires skill and affection.
A scientist and artist you will be,
And a full measure of satisfaction you will see.

John G. Bruhn

Preface

Several years ago, I was given an assignment to complete a paper on an issue associated with the nursing profession. The dynamic faculty facilitator, Dr. Ellen Fahy, assessed the paper in relation to creativity of presentation and content. That assignment continues to be one of the most valuable assignments that I completed in my early nursing career. Creativity was a new concept to me at the time. The assignment was challenging and stimulating because it encouraged me to think creatively. Since that time, creativity and creative problem solving are an integral part of my personal and professional life. It is with great enthusiasm that I introduce nurses to these vital concepts.

The ideas presented in this volume can be helpful to nurses in many roles. Creativity is not reserved for a specific group. It defies the barriers that delineate one role from another. Therefore, this volume is written for all nurses who are eager to increase their creative potential.

The creative problem-solving process is not a unique methodology for nursing. It is used by many professions to successfully solve problems. The five step process is congruent with nursing process. It is a deliberative problem-solving methodology which encourages creativity and creative production. The interdisciplinary nature of the process makes it very useful and applicable to the health professions.

This volume is an outcome of many years of service devoted to the development of creative behavior of individuals. Frank and I have presented workshops for many professional and lay groups; the exercises in this book are an outgrowth of these workshops. Much of the inspiration for the workshops evolved from our long association with the Annual Creative Problem Solving Institute at Buffalo, New York. The fantastic voluntary faculty of the Institute provides an annual immunization to keep our creative instincts alive.

The topic of creativity is lightly interspersed in the nursing literature. It is amazing that creativity has not been consistently and vigorously pursued by the nursing leadership. Therefore, in this book we emphasize the importance of creativity and place it in proper perspective. It is not too late to make creativity a common characteristic of nurses. The profession will be changed dramatically by the contributions that creative nurses can make. The time is ripe for creativity to flourish.

Shirley Steele, RN, PhD

Prologue

Throughout the history of mankind, there has been a great emphasis placed on having a healthy body. Even ancient Greeks stressed a healthy body-healthy mind concept. The assumption was made that if the body was healthy, the mind would be healthy also.

Contemporary society also places great importance on maintaining a healthy body. Note the Olympics, the sports programs, the physical leisure programs in order to validate this fact. All of these activities are geared to keep the body healthy so it can function effectively. At the same time, there are dietary or nutritional programs offered to compliment the physical fitness programs. These programs prescribe what, how, and when to eat in order to keep the body in top physical condition. A program that should probably be promoted is a new program that focuses on developing the mind, as the mind influences significantly what happens to the body. We need to awaken our minds, with mental gymnastics, to rid ourselves of sloppy thinking. This book focuses on how to improve the mind in order to think more creatively. It is a program for self-improvement. This book should serve to stimulate, challenge, and provoke you to look at yourself and the environment around you in a different light. Thinking creatively is a way of life. Creative thinking can result in a positive change in behavior. Many benefits can accrue to individuals and to society as a result of these changes in human behavior.

The exercises in this volume may seem like play on first inspection. This analogy is correct, as almost all creativity involves purposeful play. The play-like qualities of the activities make them useful as well as enjoyable to complete. However, the playful qualities should not encourage the reader to proceed through the exercises too quickly. The unleashing of creative potential takes some time to complete. The time factor is determined by the job that needs to be done. Some persons have nurtured their creativity and imagination throughout their lives. These exercises will add to their repertoire of useful techniques for keeping their creativity alive, well, and growing. Others will find themselves digging out from under layers and layers of protective covering that discouraged creative expression. In these instances, creativity will emerge at a slower, more painful pace. The main thing to keep in mind is not to get discouraged. No one has a monopoly on creative behavior. It can be owned by everyone. The exercises are designed as challenges that can be met. They are not a test of intelligence. Many intelligent people are lacking in expression of creativity. So proceed through the exercises as though you are a child enthralled by living each day to its fullest. Play awhile. Rest awhile. Return frequently. You will increase your curiosity and delight in living. You will wonder if our "solutions" are reasonable. You will see new "solutions" that are far greater than the ones provided in the discussions. But, most importantly, you have the opportunity to mobilize your inner resources to become a more alive, exciting person—a person who can transfer the excitement generated from the exercises to life situations that require new perspectives in thinking to enhance the decision-making process. Research clearly shows that actively pursuing play-like activities increases creative productivity. You have the innate potential to expand your imagination, increase your curiosity, and participate in discovery. Begin now to use the exercises to bring out your creative qualities that are certain to bring new excitement to your personal and professional life.

Table of Contents

Part I

Backround Information

Encounters in Thinking Creatively

Scenario

A long time ago there was a remote island located in the South Pacific that was inhabited by a group of people. One day the people were alerted to a radio broadcast that indicated the island would be destroyed by an approaching typhoon of 150 miles per hour winds and a tidal wave of over 50 feet high. The island was only 10 feet above the sea. There was no escape from the typhoon's destruction. The leader of the island gathered the people together to determine what they should do for the remaining 24 hours each had left on this earth...

Mental and emotional stress causes disease. Stress throws the body off balance. Thinking creatively can help to restore the emotional and physical integrity of the body. Stress or anxiety is thinking that is out of control. Many people are confined in mental institutions because their thinking is out of balance with reality. They believe that they are someone else or that someone is after them. These individuals stretch their imagination and are unable to re-establish reality. Thinking creatively is a potential aid to help individuals cope with stress in a positive manner. Thinking creatively is good therapy for preventing illness. Mental and emotional stresses subside when an individual looks at problems in a constructive manner.

Important elements that separate human beings from other animals are the ability to think and to reason. As human beings, we think a great deal even though we are frequently unconscious of our thinking process. In our daily lives, we spend a considerable amount of time thinking. We think while we are awake and while we are asleep. Although we may not realize it, our dreams are part of our thinking process. All thinking is not creative in nature. It is unnecessary to be creative 100% of the time. For example, answering a ringing phone does not require us to think creatively, but it does require us to think. We spend time thinking in an attempt to bring order out of disorder.

In his book *Applied Imagination*,[1] Alex Osborne states that humans have four basic mental powers: *absortive*—the ability to observe and to apply attention; *retentive*—the ability to memorize and recall; *reasoning*—the ability to analyze and to judge; and *creative*—the ability to visualize, foresee, generate ideas, and be imaginative. Through the first two mental powers, individuals learn and through the last two, they think. While we all think most of the time, however, thinking creatively is not a major part of that thinking. It is acceptable to step out from the conventional logical mind to resolve a problem. Developing our minds to think creatively is an excellent resource for solving problems or conflicts. Creative thinking is a change in behavior for some individuals. Thinking creatively can make a positive difference in one's attitude and outlook not only when facing problems but also when coping with other life situations. A positive outlook or optimistic view of sensing situations is indicative of healthy behavior. A person who thinks creatively is in a much better position to cope with the process of change on a day-to-day basis. Change is a way of life and coping with it creatively is a constructive way to deal with change.

The individual mind is very powerful. Each person is capable of creative thought, but through many years of environmental and cultural conditioning, people have not been encouraged to think creatively. We tend to act the way others expect us to act.

There are four basic states of thinking:

1) Vertical or Sequential—the expected
2) Lateral—the unexpected
3) Creative—the novel
4) The 4th dimension—the unexplainable

The first state of thinking, *vertical,* is the type of thinking that is expected of us. This thinking approach seems to be the "right way" to think. It is a logical and progressive thought process based on a sequence of steps or building blocks of thinking. Vertical thinking is not wrong; however, it sometimes prevents us from solving a conflict by stifling the flow of ideas. Vertical thinking is similar to constructing an electric motor from a set of drawings. All of the parts must be assembled in a prescribed sequence in order to make the motor operate safely. This type of thinking is logical (expected) and each part that is assembled is built upon the preceding part. Vertical thinking is the prevailing mode of an individual's thinking effort.

Vertical thinking is a stepwise process. Each step must be correct at each stage and each thinking step selects and concerns itself with only what is pertinent.

The second state of thinking is called *lateral* thinking, that is, thinking the unexpected. Lateral thinking, popularized in Edward DeBono's books,[2,3] expands the ability to think in new directions. This thinking process breaks the habit of logical or vertical thinking and opens the mind to creative thoughts. An essential element of lateral thinking is that it is not sequential. It does not have to be correct at each stage like the process of vertical thinking. It is not restricted to relevant or available information. An individual can move from one piece of information to another, bypassing some elements and filling in this information later. General George Patton, in World War II, used this approach in winning many battles. Instead of capturing town after town in a sequential manner, he bypassed many of them and returned later. By that time, the towns were cut off from their resources and were easier to capture. The purpose in using lateral thinking is to enhance the possibility of discovering a new and different approach to solving a problem.

The third state of thinking is *creative* thinking. Thinking creatively is not vertical or sequential thinking even though creativity does recognize the value of this kind of thinking. If it is true that we use only 10% of our potential, then it is also true that only a small percentage of our potential is involved in thinking creatively. Thinking creatively is a significantly different thought process even though it is not fully understood. This type of thought process adds a third dimension to the process of thinking. Whereas, vertical thinking is in one direction and lateral thinking in several directions, in a two-dimensional plane, thinking creatively adds a third direction or plane. Thinking creatively stretches the mind in order to use its imagination. It is the eureka stage of the thinking process. While much of vertical thinking is based upon past experiences, creative thinking goes beyond past experiences to resolve situations.

Lateral thinking helps an individual to be more effective in thinking creatively. It pushes a person to move beyond the expected and unexpected to find innovative solutions. Creative thinking opens up vistas that appear to come from nowhere. It is important to realize that an individual must be knowledgeable in an area to see the possibilities and make the connections that are possible in vertical thinking. Anything is possible within a creative mind. Jules Verne, who wrote *20,000 Leagues Under The Sea,* once remarked that "whatever one man is capable of conceiving, other men will be able to achieve." Put another way; whatever the mind can conceive, an individual can achieve.

The fourth state of thinking (for lack of a better description) is called the *4th Dimension* of thinking. This thinking is cosmic; it is holistic. Scientific data, as presently known, does not support the results. It is intuitive, a sixth sense or high energy level between people and things. It's a Gestalt: the sum is greater than its parts. Some people call it extrasensory perception (ESP). This area of thinking or sensing is a source of continuing controversy. Many psychologists are divided in their thinking regarding this issue. Some psychologists believe in it, while others remain unconvinced of its existence.

Extrasensory perception can be divided into five areas:[5]

1) Telepathy—thought transference from one person to another.

2) Clairvoyance—the ability to perceive objects or events without the use of the senses.

3) Precognition—ability to perceive a future event.

4) Deja vu—the illusion that one has previously had a given experience.

5) Psychokinsis (PK)—a mental operation that affects an object or an energy system.

How many times have you gone to a party, a meeting, or some type of gathering and gravitated towards an individual or group and then discovered that you shared a common bond? Maybe the stranger went to the same school, or knew a friend of yours, or the topic he or she was discussing was of great interest to you. "It's a small world, isn't it?" Some people consider this chance encounter a mere coincidence. But is it? What is the driving force or reason that attracted you to that individual or group? Was this a 4th-dimension state of thinking/sensing between you and the encounter?

Although this area of thinking is highly controversial because we do not have the support data nor instruments to measure this phenomena of thinking, it is best at this time to withhold judgment until more information is available. It must be remembered that, once, people thought the earth was flat, the sun revolved around the earth, and going to the moon was impossible; these ideas were not destroyed until some human mind opened the way for developing new technology. If we listened to the vertical thinker, the expected kind of thinking that provided the experts with no surprises, we would not be where we are today. We would not be enjoying many of the things we presently hold in high esteem. How many times have the so-called experts been wrong?

In order to gain a perspective on the four states of thinking—*vertical, lateral, creative,* and *4th dimension*—the following example is used:

> The energy situation that confronts the world is immensely complex. To resolve this situation, a person thinking *vertically* would tend to find oil by putting all of his/her efforts into drilling one well. In this way, the vertical thinker attempts to drill the same hole deeper and deeper, proceeding very rigidly along the route with the highest probability. This kind of thinking is based largely upon utilizing past experiences.
>
> The person thinking *laterally* probably attempts to drill several wells in different geographical locations in his/her search to discover oil.
>
> The person thinking *creatively* might attempt to find a solution to the energy problem by studying the effect of the waves, tides, winds, solar system, etc, and by disregarding oil wells altogether.
>
> The *4th-dimensional* thinker uses the dividing rod or forked stick to locate the oil. The results of the 4th-dimensional thinker are better than random or chance.

In order for the reader to better understand, appreciate, and experience some of these different thinking states, the following activities are presented. You should try them first by yourself and later, if possible, with others. At first you may feel uncomfortable, as a change in your thinking occurs, but be assured that as you develop this skill in thinking creatively, the benefits are very rewarding.

ACTIVITIES/EXPERIENCES

1. Draw a circle, any size and place a dot in it.
2. Draw a circle to represent a pie. Divide this pie into 8 pieces.
3. Note the two lines drawn in Fig. 1. What do you observe? Record the information. Note the two lines in the second drawing. Record your observation.
4. Take six wooden matches (they could be straws, or toothpicks) and make four equilateral triangles out of these six matches. No bending or breaking of the matches is allowed.

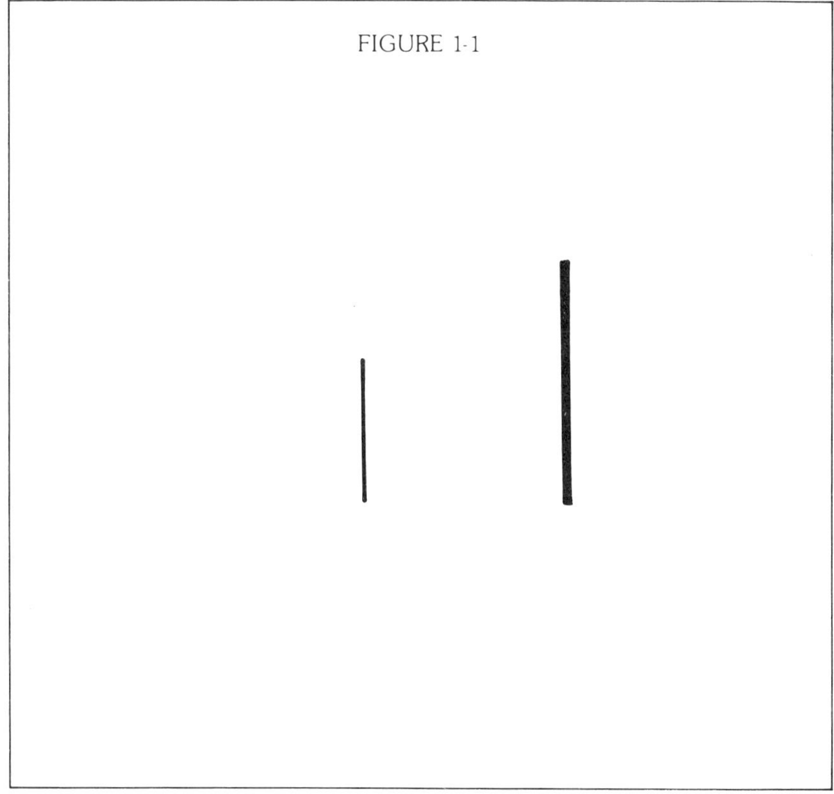

FIGURE 1-1

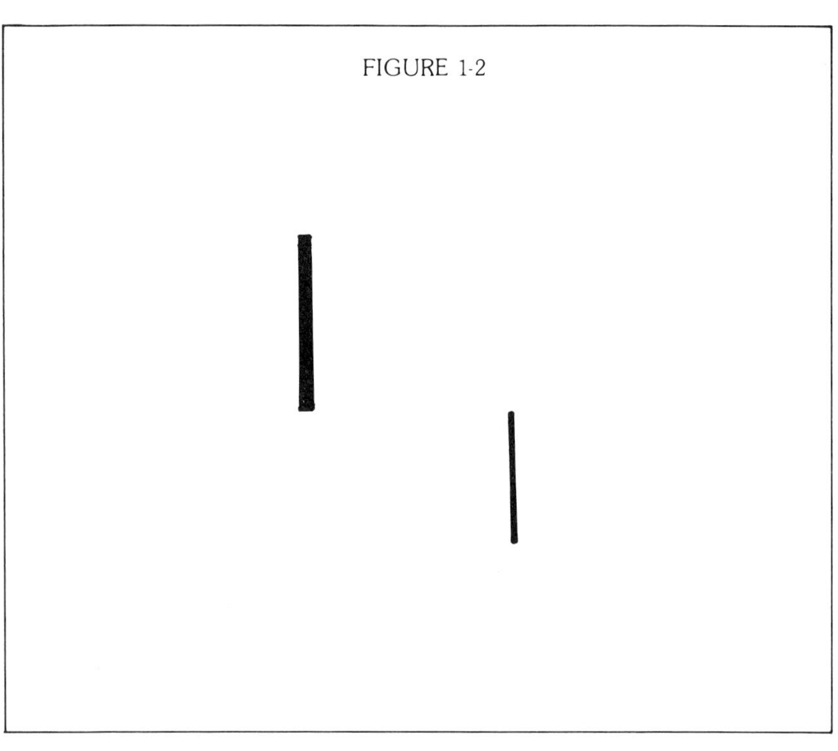

FIGURE 1-2

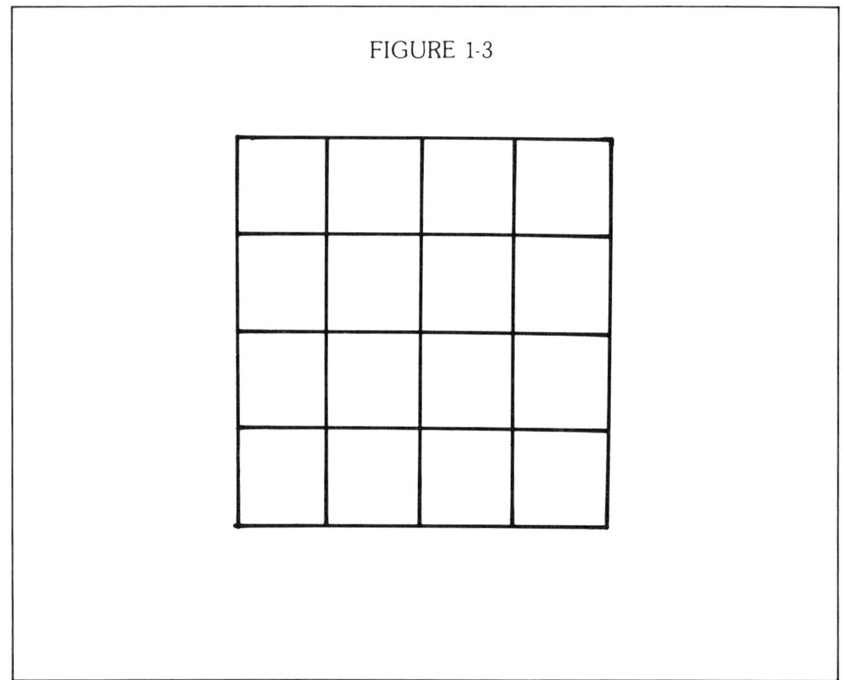

FIGURE 1-3

5. Count the number of squares you see as you view Fig. 1-3. Place this number on a sheet of paper and then ask others how many they see. Try to have a group consensus and record the number of squares.

6. Connect all nine dots in Fig. 1-4 with four straight lines without removing your writing instrument or retracing any line. For those who might be familiar with this problem do it with only three straight lines. To further stretch the mind, connect all nine dots with only one straight line. It can be done!

EXPLANATIONS

1. Most vertical thinkers place the dot in the center. The dot can be placed anywhere within the circle.

2. Did you divide the pie in eight equal pieces? Why? The directions did not tell you to do so. Vertical and habitual thinking is occurring. Another way of solving the situation is found in Fig. 1-5.

3. You would probably record some of the following information: there are two lines, they are parallel, one is wider than the other, they are black lines, etc. But what if you are told that the lines are fence posts? Now what do you see and observe? Your imagination now puts depth into the picture as a perspective drawing so that one fence post is closer than the other. Now both lines (fence posts) appear to be the same size because your mind has

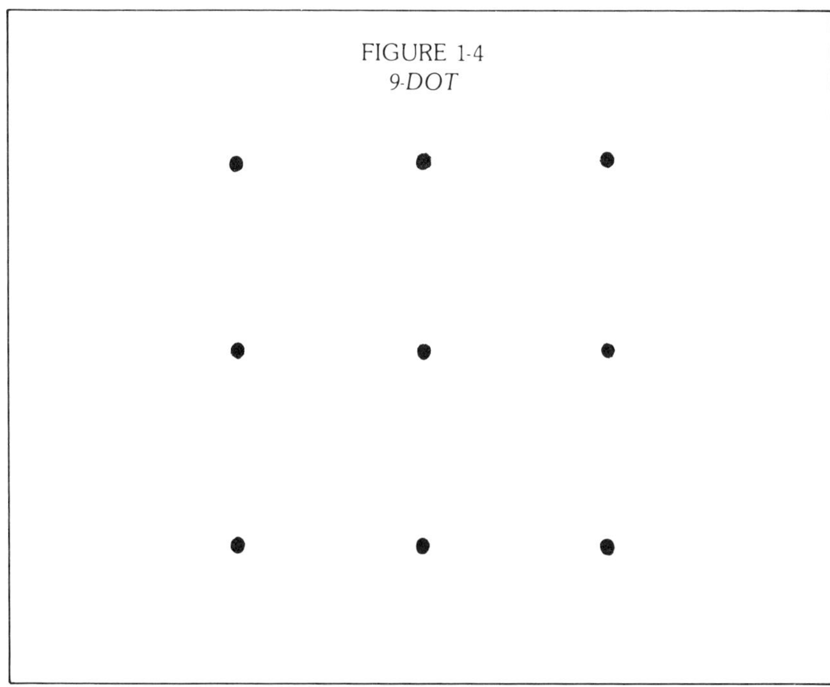

FIGURE 1-4
9-DOT

visualized them in perspective. The same can be said about the other two lines except that the mind places the fence posts in different perspective. What must the mind do to see these two lines (posts) as the same height? One is seen on a hill or mound for the first post. See Fig. 1-6.

4. One solution is a pyramid. One must move from a two-dimensional plane to a three-dimensional one. Rarely will the vertical thinker free his/her mind into the third dimension in this situation. The individual usually begins by using three matches to construct one triangle and then tries in vain to form the three triangles with the other three matches. The solution is not obtained by most people. Another solution in one plane is shown in Fig. 1-7.

5. Vertical thinkers tend to use their logical mind and add up the squares in a sequential manner. The first total would be 16, then 17 (the 16 are enclosed in one large square). Lateral thinkers see the 17 plus they see groups of four squares making a larger square, then groups of three squares making a larger square for a total of 30 if viewed in a two-dimensional plane. Using this problem with groups in which individuals had previously recorded their number of squares observed indicated two important factors. First, in most group concensus, the number of squares observed is usually larger than individual efforts. This indicates that, on most problem-solving tasks, group effort produces a more workable solution than an individual working on the

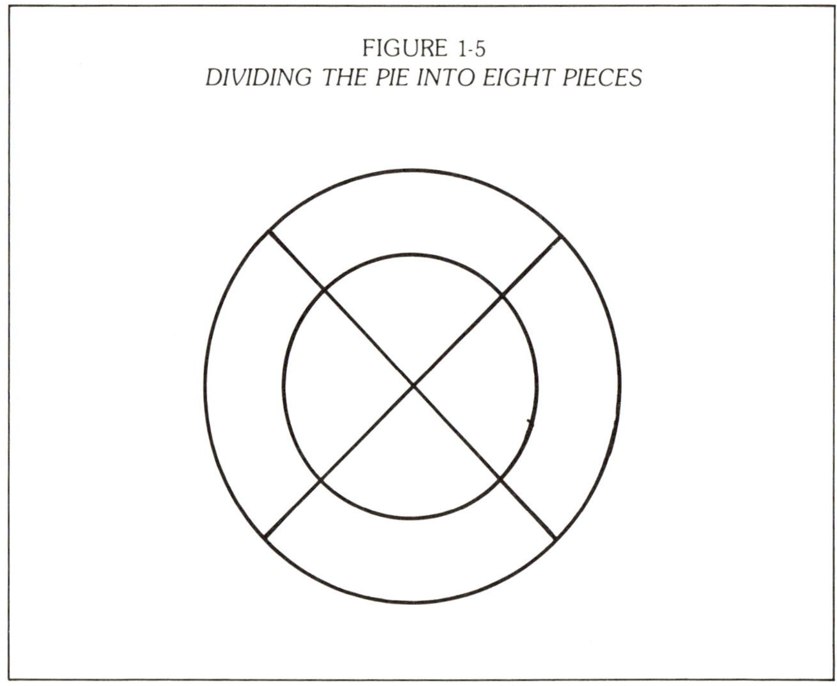

FIGURE 1-5
DIVIDING THE PIE INTO EIGHT PIECES

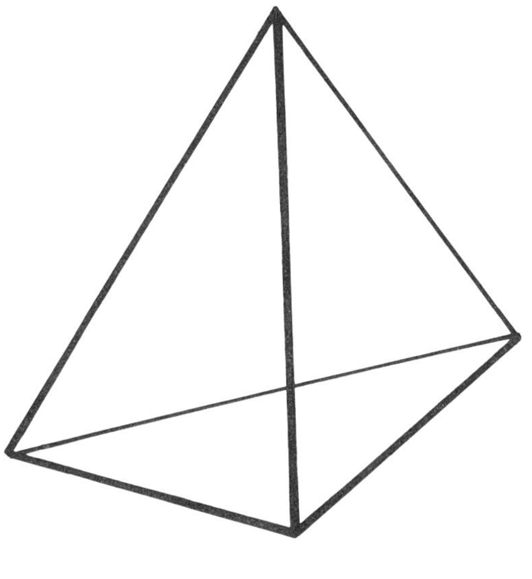

FIGURE 1-6
FOUR EQUILATERAL TRIANGLES (THREE-DIMENSIONAL)

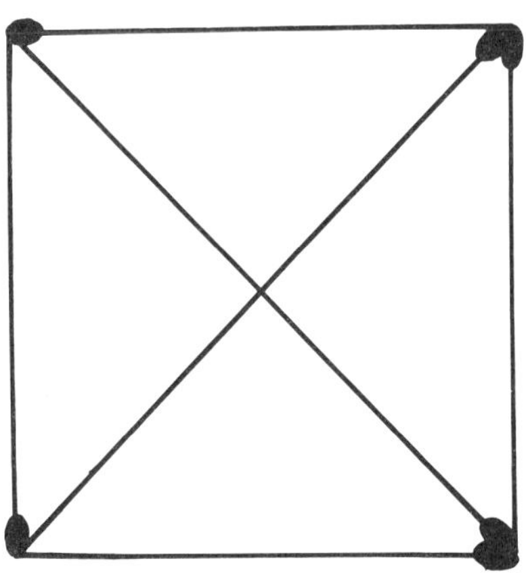

FIGURE 1-7
FOUR EQUILATERAL TRIANGLES (IN ONE PLANE)

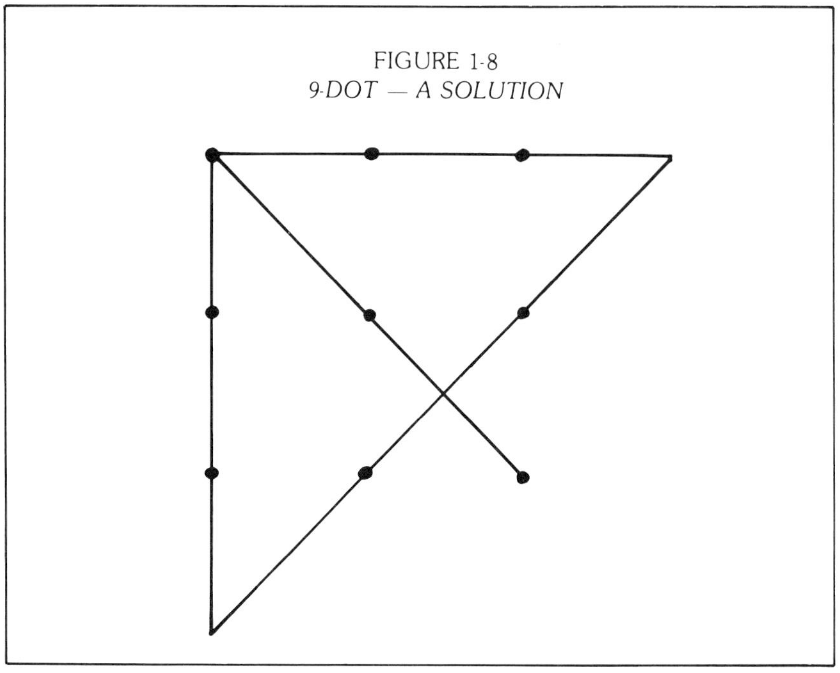

same problem. Studies prove that group efforts are superior in their thinking ability over individual efforts whether the problem involved creative abilitity, judgment, or both. Also, as you increase the number of possibilities, the superiority of the group over individual responses increases. The possible reason for this is that the available knowledge towards the solution of the problem is increased due to the interaction of the minds.

If, for example, three individuals, each representing different backgrounds and experiences, are brought together to engage a problem, certain elements are evident. First, there are experiences or backgrounds that are common to all three persons. However, there are areas that might be shared with two members of the group and not with the other member. But, there is a larger area in each person's background and experience that is not shared. It is usually from this area of knowledge and experience in group dynamics that a synergistic solution (creative) may occur. The creative thinker sees an infinite number of squares. By adding another dimension, it is viewed as a set of blocks in a wall.

The 4th-dimensional thinker has many interpretations.

6. This is an example of "boxed-in" thinking. Vertical thinkers have great difficulty in solving this problem because they tend to stay within or are "boxed" by the nine dots. This is also a cultural block in our thinking process. An Eskimo has very little trouble solving this situation. The solution(s) to the

problem is to move out beyond the nine dot area. ONE solution using four lines is presented in Fig. 1-8.

The above activities attempt to demonstrate some of the different states of thinking that most individuals experience. Becoming aware of these different thought processes is an important first stage in creative thinking. Using this awareness in solving problems or conflicts in a creative manner is the second stage. The creative approach to solving problems is different than just "solving" problems. By removing some of the mystery, magical, supernatural, or "for genius only" concepts, thinking creatively can be part of everyone's life. One doesn't have to be a Michelangelo, Jonas Salk, or Marie Curie to think creatively. One does not have to be an artist, writer, or sculptor to be creative or to have creative thoughts. Thinking creatively is used in a person's personal as well as in his/her professional life. It can also be used in solving society's ills. It is imperative to recognize the different kinds of thinking and different processes involved in creative thinking as compared to the processes used to acquire knowledge.

The brain is a complex organ. It has three main functions: to feel and receive input; to think and associate the input; and to remember or to develop memory ability. The ability to think creatively can be enhanced by reading, experiencing, sharing, possessing a positive outlook, a questioning attitude, visualizing, avoiding placing too many constraints on a given situation, talking, observing, synthesizing, etc. In other words, thinking creatively is being open to a variety of inputs! The individual who has a closed mind and suffers from intellectual myopia will not be likely to think creatively. In order to be competent in creative thinking ability, it is necessary to develop confidence and to value creativity as a positive force in our lives.

People who think creatively tend to be happy people who make things happen. People who pretend to think are more passive people who relate to things that happen to other people. People who do not think tend to be stressful people who have limited knowledge of what is happening. Whatever greatness has been achieved in our world, there is more to come through the use of our creative thinking powers.

> ......*If you remember at the beginning of this chapter, there was a story about a south sea island being hit by a typhoon. One suggestion that was made to the leader was to bring everybody together and have a party. If one was to die, one should die eating and drinking. Another suggestion was to have the people gather together and pray to the gods. If they were to die, they needed to atone for their sins. A third suggestion was made by an individual who would have no part of the first two suggestions. He was going to the library to read some books in order to discover how to live under water. Did someone think creatively?*

Chapter 2

Creative Thinking: Using Both Sides of the Brain

The concept that the brain is divided into two different modes of thinking has been around for centuries. Its origin can be traced back to Hippocrates in 400 B.C. when he identified the two hemispheres within the brain. Since 1970, there has been extensive brain research focused on both the physical and psychological sides of the brain. A great amount of credit to present investigations and research in this duality of brain thinking is owed to Dr. Roger Sperry and his work on "split brain surgery." The implications seem to direct that each hemisphere is unique in its operation—each side of the brain is capable of unique thinking powers. It is important to make clear at this point that no attempt is made to advocate that one side of the brain is more important than the other side of the brain. Both sides of the brain need to be used to their fullest advantages. In other words, while the use of one side of the brain may be better for achieving a specific task, there is a need to use both halves of the brain for creative thinking to emerge.

Basically, the brain can be said to have two "minds." The cerebral cortex of the brain is divided into two hemispheres (right and left) that is connected by the corpus callosum. The left hemisphere controls the right side of the body while the right hemisphere controls the left side of the body. The two hemispheres tend to specialize in different cognitive functions even though both sides of the brain tend to share the potential that is within the brain (see Fig. 2-1). In most people, both halves of the brain participate in most states of thinking. The left side of the brain is sometimes called the logical part of the brain. Its operation seems to process information in a logical, deductive, sequential manner such as in vertical thinking (Chapter 1). The left side of the brain seems to be well-adapted in verbal, auditory, mathematical and convergent function. The right hemisphere is capable of holistic thinking, can synthesize information better, recognizes faces, is more intuitive (knowledge without recourse to inference) as compared to the logical left side of the brain. The right side of the brain is more emotional in that it operates on a sense of "feeling" of what is happening within a situation. This "feeling" or intuition is making connections without going through a series of steps; the emphasis is on the perception of the whole situation. A Gestalt. The right hemisphere is more visual, musical, spatial, divergent, inductive and creative in its functions.

Medical research has confirmed that the brain has these two areas of specialization. Clinical cases have indicated that left-hemisphere damage in patients results in impaired language ability. A right-hemisphere brain damage may not interrupt the speech of a person, but it does cause problems in spatial awareness, musical ability, or in recognizing people.

This duality of the brain helps us better understand behavior. Many times our intellect (the logical side) suggests a course of action while the other side (the intuitive) indicates a feeling that we should do something else. In this situation, both sides of the brain are working within the individual in order for that person to make a better decision.

In western culture, it is safe to assume that we are or have been mostly a left-hemisphere society. Our schools emphasize the three R's (Reading, 'Riting and 'Rithmetic). This is one reason why we are left-hemisphere oriented. The rewards for promotion in school are based upon logical and rational behavior. Hopefully, this unilateral emphasis on left brain orientation, within our schools, is changing.

It is quite possible that we have been using the words "right" and "wrong" in solving problems incorrectly. Maybe we should use "right" and "left" to explain why a solution to a problem can or cannot work. It would seem that in our society we have had a preponderance of the left-brain thinking to solve many of our problems. There is a need to balance this left-thinking with more right-brain thinking.

Scientists, attorneys, mathematicians, police, and judges' are involved in logical and sequential type of thinking. Artists, sculptors, designers, writers, architects, and decision makers tend to be more right-hemisphere oriented. They sometimes appear to be irrational in their behavior because they do not conform to the so-called "norm."

Although both hemispheres are similar in structure, we need to take advantage of their specialization or functions. It is important to emphasize that it is not a split brain but rather that it is a unified whole with specialized parts. If the left half of the brain is superior in language as compared to the right side, the left half will be used for languages as often as possible. If the

FIGURE 2-1*	
HEMISPHERIC DOMINANCE	
CLINICAL AND EXPERIMENTAL EVIDENCE	
Left Hemisphere	Right Hemisphere
(Right Side of Body)	(Left Side of Body)
Speech/Verbal	Spatial/Musical
Logical, Mathematical	Holistic
Linear, Detailed	Artistic, Symbolic
Sequential	Simultaneous
Controlled	Emotional
Intellectual	Intuitive, Creative
Dominant	Minor (Quiet)
Wordly	Spiritual
Active	Receptive
Analytic	Synthetic, Gestalt
Reading, Writing, Naming	Facial Recognition
Sequential Ordering	Simultaneous Comprehension
Perception of Significant Order	Perception of Abstract Patterns
Complex Motor Sequences	Recognition of Complex Figures

Trotter RJ: The other hemisphere. Science News 109:219, 1976.

right half is better able to perceive abstract patterns than the left, it will predominate. What is significant is that each half of the brain can process both kinds of materials; it is simply not efficient to act in this matter.

In presenting information to others, most people tend to start at the top of the paper or chalkboard and list the material downward in a sequential manner. People who make outlines for their writing or other activities also do this. This giving and recording of information is basically a left-brain function. In order to change to a right-brain operation, a different method for presenting and recording information is necessary. Instead of starting at the top of the chalkboard or sheet of paper, start recording in the center of the writing area such as a box, circle, ellipse, or some geometric form. From this enclosed area, additional information can be presented or recorded to radiate in many directions. It does not have to be recorded in a spoke wheel array but can be recorded in random fashion. There is no exactness as to what is placed where but drawing a line and lettering the information on the line has advantages over traditional longhand writing. By using creative key words, retention of the information is increased. Also, as one needs to add information, it can be added without the same concern as there might be in an outline form.

Designers who are right-brain thinkers rather than left-brain thinkers use this method to generate and record information. Also, they use graphics as well as words to communicate their thoughts. The ability to remember or recall information is increased because of the lettering and positioning on the paper.

If we accept the hypothesis that the brain separates its functions or operations into what each part performs best, we should be able to maximize the individual's potential. Although there has been much speculation in the area of right brain versus left, continuing interest and ongoing investigation should provide vitally needed information in our efforts to understand human behavior and how humans process problems. To increase our creative problem solving ability and to enhance thinking creatively, we must provide an environment that will stimulate both sides of the brain.

ACTIVITIES/EXPERIENCES

1. Fold your hands. Which thumb is on top? In a group exercise it would be about 50-50 as to the number who would have either their right or left thumb on top. Now reverse the position of the thumb. How does it feel? Odd, uncomfortable different, etc. These are normal reactions in this position change of the thumbs.

2. Fold your arms as you normally do. Relax. Which arm is on top? Now reverse the position of the arm. Did you have difficulty doing it? How does it feel?

3. Rotate your hands forward. Now rotate your hands backward. Now try to rotate one hand forward and the other hand backward at the same time. Most people can rotate both hands in the same direction but find it very difficult to rotate each hand in a different direction at the same time.

Research indicates that by changing to the second position of folding your arms, legs, and hands it is not only better healthwise but muscle tone and circulation will improve, and it will help stimulate use of the right side of the brain. The findings also show that people have the potential to be more productive in the use of arms, legs, and hands.

A college senior who attempted to utilize the other parts of his body supported the findings. He not only became a better athlete, was healthier, but showed a remarkable change in his approach to learning and personal growth.

4. Play some music that activates the right hemisphere. It is usually not the same kind of music that one listens to while driving a car or shopping in a store. That kind of music might be more left hemisphere for you. What is

needed is music that will relax you and stimulate the other side of the brain. The right hemisphere is usually stimulated by a different kind of music than the left side finds enjoyable.

5. For those individuals who are interested in stimulating right-hemisphere thinking, excellent tools to use, in addition to music, include: films (short, colorful); slides and posters; and the use of metaphors, symbols, abstractions, and sounds (like water flowing). If one is a teacher, parent, or adult trainer, the utilization of one or combination of the above in a given time is quite effective. Having people fantasize an experience or recall one helps develop the right hemisphere. In this manner, developing the whole brain approach is increased. Meditation is also a help in using both sides of the brain effectively.

Art, painting, sculpturing, ceramics, crafts, writing poems, etc, all help to bring about a holistic approach to thinking. What is happening in the research of human intelligence since 1970 may be the most important development in psychology since Freud.

Chapter 3

Observation and Perception

This chapter is concerned with the sensory aspects that are involved in solving problems creatively. It should be pointed out that all sensory aspects or functions—structural-mechanical, physiological, and cultural—must be incorporated. The first two, however, are more obvious and better understood as functions while the third, the cultural function, persists in being a source of confusion, discord, conflict, and apprehension. Nevertheless, our senses, although physiological, are culturally conditioned.

It is important to emphasize that we primarily sense what our culture has taught us to respond to. Sensing is a learned experience and, therefore, we can improve our ability to use our senses. It is only the rare creative individual who senses beyond this cultural conditioning. It is this person who succeeds in providing the insights which alter a culture. These insights, in turn, become a part of our cultural heritage and eventually they, too, crystalize into stereotypes.

In his book *Be Careful of What You Want, You Might Get It,*[1] Leroy Schneider states that from our basic senses learning takes place as follows: 83% from sight, 11% from sound, 3 1/2% from smell, 1 1/2% from touch, and 1% from taste. We retain 10% from reading, 20% from hearing, 30% from seeing, and 50% from combining hearing and seeing. See Fig. 3-1. From this data it becomes clear that the more senses that are involved in the learning process, the greater is the potential to learn and retain the information we gather from life's experiences. The various senses bring the raw material to the mind. The way the mind organizes the observations is influenced by past experiences, beliefs, and attitudes.

Sight is a faculty; seeing is an art. The eyes may see every line in an observation but the mind organizes the observation into a form that is meaningful for the individual. Another individual can put a different meaning to it, however. Seeing is not merely a visual experience. Seeing is also the way a visual experience is witnessed. The differences seen in the arts and group situations result from the interpretation placed on what is seen. Looking doesn't guarantee that observation is taking place. During observation (when we look or use our senses), people become more sensitive to problems or challenges. The more that is learned through careful observation, the more a person realizes how much more there is to learn.

One of the important factors that helps to develop and bring out creativity in people is a keen sense of observation and perception. A creative problem solver's ability is enhanced by his/her accurate observations. Many of our behaviors and attitudes are the result of what we observe.

Observation as a basic human function is not new. It is as old as man. Cave drawings represent the oldest preserved observation that man has recorded. To observe things is not enough; however, observation is composed of two complex human functions: attention and perception. Two individuals can see/observe the same thing, but their perceptions or conclusions can be entirely different. It is even more difficult to get consensus when a group of people observe the same thing, using one or more of the senses. The same principle applies as well to what we hear, smell, taste, or feel. It is possible that the reason why sight is so important is that nature seems to favor sight over the other senses. Even before birth, the eyes of the fetus move. From the moment of birth to approximately eight weeks old, the infant attempts to comprehend its environment through its eyes. Some people have postulated that infants come to know physical objects as solid and tangible through visual experience and not through a reliance on touch. In our culture, we tend to be more visually oriented than a "feeling" (sensing) society. When an individual loses one sense completely or the sense is impaired, the other senses tend to become more acute in order to compensate. If sight is lost, a tactile encounter with a thorn can give as much insight into the character of the thorn as the visual perception. The human eye is the receptacle or faculty through which images pass. It is the opening or gateway to the brain. The same can be said of the skin. It provides the tactile stimulation impulses to the brain. Attention to a sense response results in the opening or releasing of the gate. Observation is the welcoming in of the stimuli, and perception is what the brain registers in response to the stimuli.

Most humans are endowed with the ability to observe. It can be honed or dulled by our emotions without our knowing it. It is necessary that good observation be kept sharp because it is the basis for intelligent decisions. Good observation plus imagination equals good ideas. Good observation helps us to gather facts in order to find the real problem. Good observation also helps us in selling the idea to others. Good observations are necessary in order to have good perceptions.

What is observation? It is a mental skill. To observe is to take notice, to show attention, to be alert, to scrutinize carefully, to inspect for detail, to be cognizant, to recognize, or to contemplate. As with any skills, keen observation can be and must be learned. The degree of perfection attained is related to the amount of time spent practicing the art. The skill of increasing our observation takes effort, energy, and time. Although observation is a mental skill, our minds frequently distort what we observe.

Some people believe that the problems we have in observation and creativity are mental and are not within the sense organs. In this chapter, we are assuming that a person is using his/her unimpaired senses. Color blindness, hearing loss, loss of taste or smell, etc, are not included in the discussion, but these physical disabilities render problems in our attention, observation, and perception.

Attention is the time given to observe. Attention is influenced by both internal and external factors. Individual interests, desires, and motivation help determine attention and attention spans. People who are curious or inquisitive are responsive to opportunities for creating needed change. They see the possibility to improve the present situation and are not satisfied with the "status quo." Their attention may vary because they are always looking for something that will help them grow. Because they are open-minded, they are able to observe more. Some people are content with the way things are. These people usually are not very good observers and tend to resist change. Their attitude is that "it has been seen before or done before." Therefore, they believe, there is no need to spend the time needed to do it differently or better. People who are too content or not committed in a given situation usually are not effective observers.

Individuals who are action oriented tend to increase attention-effectiveness. They are better observers of past experiences and are continually looking for better ways to achieve. In this manner, their attention span is increased. Their observation power is enhanced because the brain receives more stimuli and can make more connections. When interest is high, attention is increased. An individual who recognizes an opportunity will increase personal attention given to it. Observational power is very high under these circumstances.

Perception is the process by which a person becomes aware of stimuli. Human beings become aware of stimuli through their five senses. As all humans are different, interpretations of what is perceived vary. Perception is a process within the brain that separates it from observation. It should be noted that the differences between perception and sensations are signals from our senses. They are not the same. Our senses send signals to our brains and our perceptions translate these signals, hopefully, into something meaningful.

The patterns supplied by the senses are different for each individual. The first important determinant is that no two people have the same mental and physical characteristics. Another point is that people select things that are of interest to them and ignore those things that are not of interest. And, finally, we can be misled by our expectations or past experiences. This is an attempt by the mind to make coherent what is being observed through some stimuli. We receive new stimuli and it is automatically associated with previous stimuli and may lose some of its meaning in the process. Ross Mooney,[2] who has done extensive work in observation and perception, states "perception is a prediction not a truth."

Persons need to be involved in information processing activities. This activity necessitates stimuli to be continually introduced so that the person is able to interpret the stimuli and to make meaning out of life. Healthy, motivated persons who do not receive an adequate supply of stimuli witness a sense of discomfort that leads them to seek additional perceptual information by creating it internally or by generating it from the external environment. Persons who receive too much stimulation develop mechanisms for turning off or shutting out the excessive stimuli that they perceive. Persons attempt to mediate and control the amount and intensity of stimuli they receive in order to be able to create an exciting and comfortable environment in which to live. The attending to or shutting out of selected stimuli is an important function of the human mind. Under ordinary circumstances, the mind is effective in maintaining this gatekeeper function. However, in times of stress, complicated social or environmental conditions, the mind can be faulty in this function. For instance, an infant that is reared in an overcrowded home with many adults and other children continually overstimulating him/her may learn to cut out all stimuli in an attempt to maintain equilibrium. As a result, the infant receives too little perceptual input for development to proceed. Another example is a client in an intensive care unit. The over-abundance of light and sound stimuli results in perceptual confusion and disorientation, proof that the mind is unable to adjust to the change in perceptual input.

Many errors in our perceptions are due to illusions, a mental recording of a false impression, of what is being observed. These illusions can be physical conditions such as injury to the eye, fatigue, color blindness, etc. Illusions can also be caused by a total unanalyzed impression. Habit and familiarity can also cause illusions. Many of you who have taken psychology courses or have read books in this area have seen the Ames' House. In that particular situation, the dog appears bigger than the man. An ice cube placed on a person's neck can cause a hot rather than a cold sensation. The senses can be fooled. Also, our perception of movement can be altered. The sun appears to move faster at sunset than when it is overhead. In one case, it is near a horizontal line and in the other situation it has no reference point. Every person has witnessed the sensation while sitting in a stopped car or train, that the car or train was moving while in reality it was another car or train that was actually moving. If you were the driver of the stopped car, you tended to apply the brakes because you thought you were moving.

A trapezoidal window, used by psychologists, suggests to the viewing people that it is oscillating (going back and forth) when in reality it is turning in a 360° circle. The illusion suggests that the windows have thickness, the panes are the same size, etc, when actually they are not. These illusions are caused because our past lifetime experiences are so entrenched that they actually overcome the real situation.

If our experience plays a vital role in our ability to perceive, it is equally important in dealing with people. Many times we are puzzled by the fact that others do not or cannot see a situation as we do. However, we now have a better understanding as to why they do not perceive the situation as we do—their past experiences have been different from ours; therefore, their assumptions and personal involvements are different. Isn't this an explanation for the many problems that we have in human relations? A manager may see a situation one way and those working for him/her see it quite differently.

Observation and perception is a mental skill that can be improved. The following are some ways to improve observation:

1. Be selective and observe what is important. No individual can be expected to observe everything. Select clean-cut objects to observe and know what is significant and what is insignificant.

2. Know what to look for. Because observation requires attention, a good observer must be interested in what is pertinent. A good observer does his/her homework. The more knowledgeable a person is in a particular area, the better his/her observations and perceptions can be.

3. An individual must practice observing and be checked on the correctness of his/her observations. Evaluation of the observations in relation to the results achieved is very important.

4. As a creative person, keep an open mind. Try to be aware of many possibilities. It is natural to see only what one wants to see and this must be kept in check.

5. Do not be satisfied with a general impression. It is essential that an individual makes a close examination for facts and details. A thorough analysis of a situation is very important in the decision making process.

6. Guard against habit and familiarity. As in the trapezoidal window and the stopped car, be sure that you do not see things that are not happening. Your experience can color your perception and cause you needless problems. Cultivate an inquiring mind. Wonder about things and ask the five W's—What? Where? When? Who? Why?

7. As an aid to creative problem solving, record your observations systematically. Improve your perception by making notes; keeping a diary or files help to improve a person's perception.

8. Develop a check list. If you do not know what to look for then your observations may prove futile. Preparation of a check list helps an

individual to observe what is important and what is nonessential.

And, finally, an important question to be asked in the area of observation and perception is, "Are there sensory differences between the male and female?" Are women or men superior in sensory awareness? If so, are they significant and what are the effects on thinking creatively or solving problems? There are indications that the sight sense is similar in the sexes except that males seem to have more vision defects. Males can be colorblind while it is rare for females to have this handicap. Males tend to prefer visual stimulation while females prefer auditory stimulation. Females can hear high tones better, and at least part of the time, they have a superior sense of smell. This increased sense of smell is dependent on the estrogen level in women. However, olfactory production varies cyclically with the monthly variation in estrogen production. When a woman's sense of smell decreases, her ability to taste becomes more acute. This might be an attempt by the body to compensate for the decrease in smell. It is possible that certain preconceived ideas relative to the utilization of the senses have hindered people in their career or career choices.

One of the important characteristics we have as human is the ability to change viewpoints. Changing a person's viewpoint is difficult but by sharpening our observations and thus increasing our perceptions, change can be brought about. We have learned that utilizing the senses to their greatest potential can aid us in looking at problems in a different way and that this different "looking" helps us in solving problems creatively and improving our mental health.

ACTIVITIES/EXPERIENCES

1. What is the missing number?

5	7	9	8
52	94	18	?

2. Make four nines = 100.

3. Consider three common objects such as a table, a stove and a book. What product do they suggest? What do they suggest in solving an absentee problem?

4. Without looking at your watch or timepiece, describe its face. If you drive an automobile, describe the steering wheel...the dashboard.

5. Place the letters of the alphabet that correspond to the numbers on a telephone dial. Those who have a push button dial do the same.

6. Observe the articles of clothing you are wearing. What suggestions might you make for improvement because of your observations?

7. Using a child's book, try reading it upside down. Though you might have trouble at first, with a little practice you will be able to read the words and sentences more rapidly.

8. Take pictures with a camera. Read and observe photographs, drawings, and symbols in a variety of publications.

9. Which takes up more space—a pickle or a pain? Explain why?

10. If one hand is placed in a bowl of hot water and the other in cold water, and then if both hands are placed in a bowl of tepid water, the water feels at the same time warm for one hand and cold for the other. Although we know intellectually the water cannot be cold and hot at the same time, this is how we would feel and judge it. The brain does not reject the paradox. We experience something we know to be physically impossible.

EXPLANATIONS

1. 46—the bottom number is the square of the top number in reverse.

2. 9.999 will equal 100 or $99 \frac{9}{9} = 100$.

3. In question 9 either answer (pickle-pain) can be correct. It depends upon one's interpretation.

The other exercises are self-explanatory.

Visual Perception

The following three drawings illustrate the multistability in perception. These drawings allow the viewer to perceive two or more possibilities which are different but equally as important, depending upon the experience and criteria employed by the viewer.

In Fig. 3-1, a person can view the airplane as either taking off or approaching to land. What is seen depends upon the perspective of the viewer.

In Fig. 3-2, a person can see either a rabbit or a duck. The rabbit faces the left; the duck faces the right. Because of past experience, one could be biased and see only one of the animals and not the other.

Fig. 3-3 is a drawing that is used to determine if a person can see a young girl or an old lady. Viewers of this illustration can also see a bald eagle and a porcupine. Can you see them? Perception is in the mind, not in the eyes, ears, nose, etc.

In conjunction with using these illustrations, the authors have discovered that many people have difficulty in perceiving more than one figure. This has lead to the possibility that many of these individuals resist change and many times are very opinionated. The ability to perceive and visualize is vital to the creative process. Since creativity is the putting together or making new

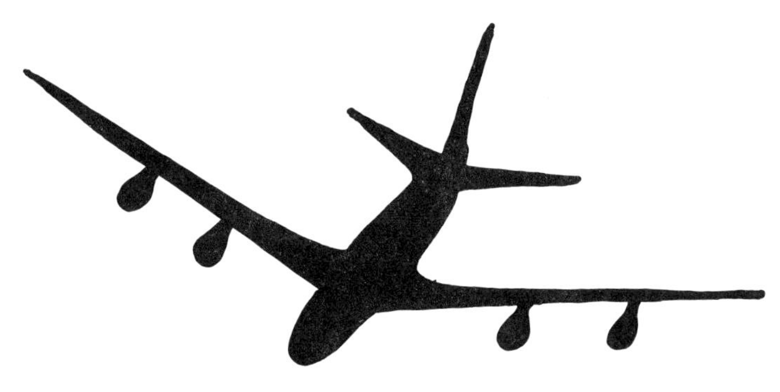

FIGURE 3-1
PLANE LANDING OR TAKING OFF?

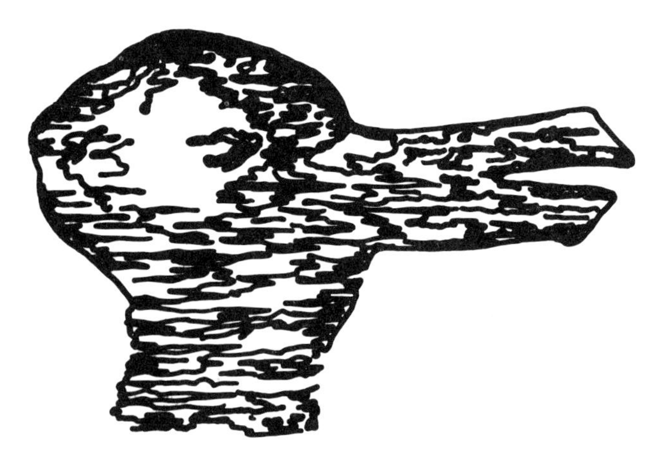

FIGURE 3-2
WHAT ANIMAL DO YOU SEE?

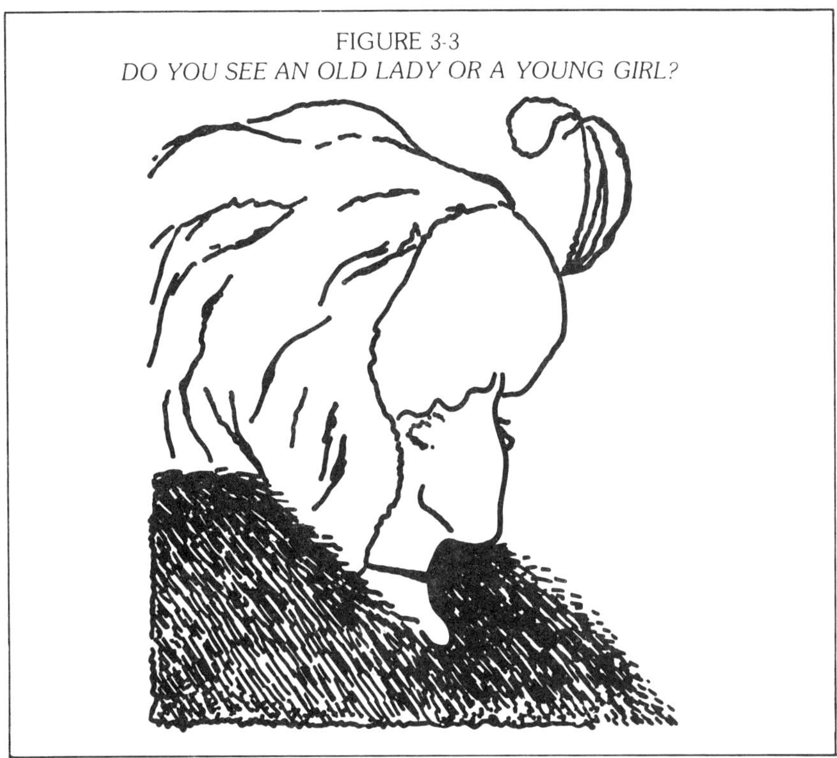

connections, the more pieces one has to work with will aid the person's perception. In relation to supervising and leading others, individuals who see only one figure are generally people who wish to continue with the "status quo." The reason might be that, while we perceive a large picture as a whole, people select only from it portions that are meaningful to them. In viewing any situation, people bring to it their past experiences, attitudes, interests, and biases. These biases and the emphasis on prior knowledge hinder people in making new connections. While many individuals might say that there is poor communication or lack of understanding, many people do not actually "see" the other possibilities in a given situation. It is important to remember that our ability to observe and perceive can be improved and sharpened, aiding us to think more creatively.

Chapter 4

Obstacles to Creative Thinking

In order for creative thinking to occur in an organization, it is important to be aware of those elements that hinder or inhibit growth of creativity. By being aware of those factors that limit people's abilities to use their minds, leaders can minimize these negative factors. The blocks to creative thinking can be classified into five categories: environmental, cultural, emotional, mental, and perceptual.

Environmental blocks are conditions within the organization or group that hinder the utilization of an individual's creative thinking. A lack of freedom in the development and exploration of new ideas to a satisfactory conclusion can inhibit future contributions by the individual. Job redundancy, boredom, and frustration coupled with stringent adherence to organizational rules are other environmental blocks to thinking creatively. In conjunction with dissatisfaction about the job, the mental attitudes of the leader limiting thinking to technical fields constrains the creative participation of the individuals. Constant surveillance by the leader indicates a lack of trust and downgrades the abilities that are possessed by individuals. Individuals who work in this environment ask themselves "Why be creative when there is no recognition given for this attribute?" In many cases where the individual is hindered in contributing his/her thoughts, group efforts can also be stifled.

One of the environmental blocks to using creative energy is the concept that persons in the group do not have any creative talent. If the leader thinks or believes that the people in the group are not creative, then the members of the group will feel the same way. If they are not recognized for having the ability to think, then they will not contribute to the workings of the organization. By this behavior the leader not only suppresses the creative talent of the group, but also the individual's imagination. When people come into this world they have an almost infinite capacity for imagining. However, our schools, social, and business organizations seem to hold back creative talent.

If there is one thing that society is sure of today it is that we are living in a world of change. Creative managers and leaders are change agents.

Managing change is a challenge not only to the manager but also to the staff. Although this may pose some problems to all parties concerned, it is important to realize that change is a way of life. A possible reason for this concern is that change usually suggests something new or different. When newness is related to creativity, the resistance to it seems to increase. We need change because it stimulates individuals and organizations to generate new ideas. Leaders must have an open mind with respect to the frequent and significant changes taking place in their organizations. Creative thinking helps leaders become more aware of their environment, more sensitive to people's needs, and more perceptive. Creative leaders are more involved with their staff—especially sharing experiences and concerns with them. They share their views rather than dictating managerial concerns, share feelings rather than talking about them, and share interpretations and extrapolations with staff when dealing with tasks and problems.

Other obstacles that hinder creative thought processes are those relating to cultural and social concerns. "Cultural blocks are social inhibitors resulting from our culture that prevent one from being his independent creative self."[1] The conformity to accepted patterns such as not wasting time on fantasy and heavy emphasis on reason and logic prevent realization of individual imagination. The analytical problem solving approach which encourages judgmental thinking stifles the individual's ability to think creatively. Conformity to this sequential left-brain thinking inhibits the possibility of divergent thinking. The culturally prevalent concept that consensus is the accepted way of life also tends to suppress independent thought and idea implementation.

Our cultural mandates, which are basically success oriented, cause frustration in individuals because failure is regarded as a stress that should not be confronted under any circumstances. Research may develop only limited innovative processes, if attempted at all, due to the negative influence of potential failure. What is actually true in the area of creativity is that stress is change and change is the opportunity for creativity to occur. Our culture discredits failure so we tend to attempt only those activities which have minimal risk of failure. The fear of "looking dumb" or "feeling inadequate," or the possibility of showing one's ignorance causes people to limit their contributions in problem solving situations to ideas that are safe and familiar.

Society assigns high value to peer pressure and behavior patterns which follow the preconceived "societal norms." Rewards are usually bestowed on those individuals who seem always to be right, to be most intelligent, and to have physical features which fit the Grecian ideals. Creative thinking and creative individuals generally do not follow these patterns; their activities, attitudes, values, and ideas are considered unacceptable and irritating and, therefore, go unrewarded. The reliance on these ill-spent values seems to gain importance as the list of academic and professional credentials increases. Many times the less creative individuals in an organization are rewarded and recognized because they do not "rock the boat." This social and organizational isolation of the creative individual is a source of anxiety and frustration to him/her.

A manager should be patient in his/her creative work force. Because there is much risk in creative endeavors, the manager should allow a greater margin for error with creative people. A willingness to take chances where he/she may be held in ridicule is an essential element of the creative individual. People such as Christopher Columbus, Henry Ford, the Wright brothers, Thomas Edison, Albert Einstein, Buckminster Fuller, T.S. Eliot, and Ernest Hemingway are individuals who were willing to take risks.

The assignment of sex roles to job descriptions limits the possibility of creative thinking. The traditional concept of masculinity is that imagination, fantasy, color, poetry, music appreciation, tenderness, romance, love of plants, cooking, household duties, and child rearing belong only in the female realm. This concept limits men from active involvement in a wide range of experiences in which they could make valuable contributions. Role constraints of female abilities is equally detrimental. Traditionally the female is associated with the nurse's role and the male with the doctor's role.

This attitude of dictating job classification based on sex hinders change and makes it seem "wrong" for a person to assume other roles. The inflexibility of our culture to regard the individual rather than the individual's gender causes much consternation and limits the potential productivity and social contributions of many people. Gradually, we are seeing women who are airplane pilots, doctors, civil engineers, and men who are nurses or are actively participating in the child rearing process.

Emotional and mental blocks to creativity, although individualized, can also be exacerbated by group pressure. Lack of self-esteem is a primary factor in the limitation of creative thought. Fear of criticism, doubt about one's creative potential, lack of self-confidence, laziness, fear of failure, excessive, uncontrolled anxiety, and basic personal insecurity all contribute to limiting creative endeavors. It is important to realize that it is impossible for a person to fail without his/her own consent. An overemphasis or preoccupation with the effects and magnitudes of life's day to day trials and tribulations leaves little or no time for the emergence of creative thinking. This all-consuming concern prejudices the way a person thinks. The inability to place these daily problems in their proper perspective can foster a negative philosophy. The individual creates mountains out of molehills and regiments his mental and physical energies into activities meant to combat problems which are actually beyond his/her control. This person exhausts his/her physical and mental powers fighting a losing battle. Self-defeated, he/she finally develops the negative attitude that whatever he attempts will fail. The creative seed is then buried in fallow ground.

A commitment to the status quo is a hindrance to creative thought even though it may appear that this is "the way to go." This sublimation of the individual's needs and drives negates all chances of developing divergent thought functions.

Compulsive individuals who may be on the verge of some neurosis are limited in their ability to express creative thought. While they may be highly imaginative, they lack the emotional balance necessary to cope with life. The creative potential can become lost in the myriad of emotions and problems. The creative thought process will, at best, be erratic in occurrence. Neurotic mechanisms can, therefore, seriously impair creative thinking.

A perceptual block to creativity is the inability to perceive situations where it is possible to be creative. This lack of insight can be found at all levels of personal and professional life. These opportunities can be the breeze which lifts the wings of creative thought over the mountains of pessimism, if only people would rely on their creative abilities and use them more readily. The breezes exist everywhere and will be found if one views problems as vehicles for creative thinking. "The perceptual blocks are those inhibitors preventing one from getting valid, relevant information from the persons, things or situations observed."[1] Rigid categorization, only seeing things as black or white, and stereotyping individuals and problems with solutions, restrict and restrain people from attempting innovative thoughts or processes.

Solving problems by only using solutions based on past experiences is a perceptual block. It does not permit one to resolve conflicts which are surfacing for the first time. This habitual attitude limits and sometimes totally shuts out innovative and imaginative possibilities.

A thorough understanding of the influences which inhibit creative thinking can minimize some of their negative effects. Unless the reason is purely pathological, studying the complexity of one's own personality and the mechanisms of the creativity/divergent thinking processes can aid in minimizing, if not totally eliminating, the effect of blocks to creativity.

Chapter 5

Techniques and Strategies for Thinking Creatively

There are many techniques and strategies that can be employed to develop creative thinking. Sometimes these can be used to produce large quantities of ideas which would not be forthcoming in an unmanaged idea-generating session. It should be noted that while one method may work well with one individual or group, it may not work well with others. Also, these idea-generating techniques can and should be used in all phases of thinking creatively in application to solving problems. These strategies require an individual to extend thinking capacities beyond past experiences which limit his/her exploration of new ideas.

The need for new and innovative ideas in patient services and research has never been greater. Creative thinking and innovation, therefore, should be developed to a high degree, should become integral parts of the nurse's formal education, and should be stressed in the daily job activities.

The following list of idea-generation techniques will assist the nurse in meeting new demands and challenges. Although this list is by no means all-inclusive, it is designed to emphasize the diversity and wide variety of techniques that are available today.

1. *Attribute listing* is a technique developed by Robert P. Crawford and described in his book *The Techniques of Creative Thinking*. The strategy is to list all the properties and/or attributes of a product or situation. Each attribute is reviewed with the intention of improving it. The evolution of the modern writing instrument can be traced to attribute listings of previous marking tools. By listing the major characteristics of the item and then analyzing each one with the idea of improving it, a synthesis of these attributes has produced the many writing devices we have today. Attribute listing is also applicable to situational conditions.

2. The *brainstorming* technique developed by Alex Osborn[2] will be discussed in depth in following chapters. The essence of brainstorming is that judgment is ruled out while ideas are being generated. Quantity of ideas is more important than quality. Wild and unusual ideas are encouraged. Hitchhiking on ideas is welcomed. Osborn's list of nine verbs—*adapt, modify, magnify, minify, substitute, rearrange, reverse,* and *combine*—is used to stimulate idea production. In conjunction with the brainstorming technique, it is possible to list the things which are

wrong with the situation. Then the group or person systematically reviews each "wrong" and suggests ways of righting it. This is called "reverse-brainstorming" and is conducted just prior to or following a "brainstorming" session. However, caution is exercised when using this technique because the negative viewpoints expressed can adversely influence the optimistic attitudes of the participants.

3. The *checklist* lists the variables, conditions, or constraints associated with a product or situation and enables a person to study the situation in its entirety. By reviewing the elements of the list, it is possible to isolate the problem or suggest improvements to the existing product or situation. Osborn's nine verbs can also be applied to this method.

4. The *collective notebook method* is a technique whereby an idea-recording book is given to each person in the problem-solving group. Daily notations are made in this book relative to the problem. These books are collected after a thirty-day period and the ideas are compiled and summarized by the group leader. The summaries are distributed to the participants. Subsequent discussions lead to the utilization of brainstorming, synectics, or other idea generation techniques to develop potential solutions to the assigned problem.

5. The *catalog-dictionary-thesaurus technique* is a random selection of two of more words from a catalog, dictionary, or thesaurus. Forcing a connection between the chosen words and the stated problem generates ideas relative to the problem. This is an excellent tool for idea generation. In addition, the use of synonyms and antonyms helps to increase the number of ideas being formulated.

6. *Forced relationships* involve the combination of ideas to produce new thoughts. While they can be used in many other techniques, forced relationships make the mind make connections which may seem irrelevant, but this stretching of the mind increases the number and quality of ideas generated.

7. *Grid and matrix analyzes* are a systematic method of examining not only alternatives but also combinations of alternatives of potential solutions. Using sliding strips which move in different directions increases the possible combinations in a given situation. While some of these combinations may seem ridiculous and impossible, the creative person may see a solution in the juxtaposition of these combinations.

8. The *gripes-complaints-improvements technique* enables a person to list factors relevant to a situation and consider them individually. Individuals closest to the situation can contribute significant ideas for improvements.

9. The *Gordon technique* is a process whereby the actual problem is

known only by the leader. The process begins with a vague problem statement, usually given in one word. Participants are encouraged to think of as many meanings as possible for the word. As the leader goes through the process, incrementally, additional information is given about the problem. This information leads to a more definitive problem which the participants are asked to solve. The individual or group is forced to make connections using all of the selected words. A spin-off of this technique is that individuals are more willing to accept the views of others and they become more open to ideas and possibilities.

The leader's strategy is to keep ideas flowing at all times. The success of this technique depends mostly on the expertise of the designated leader.

10. The *input-output method* of problem solving was developed by the General Electric Company. The identification of the goal is considered a critical point—a desired output. Once this output is clearly identified, the method moves analytically to listing possible inputs which could achieve the stated goal. When all of the inputs are listed, they are discussed, evaluated, and prioritized. The ideas are then developed into working models. This structured approach works well with people who are comfortable with logical and analytical methods of solving problems. This method still allows room for the imagination of the individuals because the technique stimulates people to discover new or alternative ways of solving the problem.

11. The *thinking big approach* is predicated on thinking big. The person is asked to imagine what might be possible if there were no constraints. He/she is to imagine, fantasize, and dream about what would be possible if unlimited resources, were available. After "thinking big," the person re-evaluates the ideas generated and then modifies them for application in the real world. This method stretches the imagination to new ideas and then tempers them for practical application.

12. The *Kepner-Tregoe method* is another of the analytical methods to problem solving whereby emphasis is on isolating the causes of the problem. It is a systematic approach to finding the "why" and "what is the cause" of the problem. The assumption made is that if you know the cause or causes, then, and only then, can you go on to the solution. This technique is especially suited to establishing "what is the problem" and the causes related to it.

13. The use of *morphological charts* is one step further in the practice of attribute listing. Morphological thinking helps a person move toward greater abstractions and hence move toward greater numbers of possibilities. Some of the basic features of a product or situation are

incorporated in the development of a new and innovative product or situation. Force fitting the relationships of the ideas is the crux of the process. By force fitting the ideas, alternative solutions are generated. The morphological change is from many alternatives generated by matrix comparison to one viable problem solution.

The procedure for this morphological chart is as follows:

a) Define the functions that must be performed by the new item/situation.

b) Using a chart, list the possible ideas for obtaining each stated function.

c) Select an idea from each function and combine the ideas for a possible solution.

The use of a morphological chart causes an individual to utilize divergent thinking, and it minimizes the influences of conventional thought processes. Another advantage is that a chart can be assembled in a relatively short period of time.[3-5]

14. The *Phillips 66 technique* was developed by Donald Phillips, a college president in Michigan. In this technique groups of six people discuss a problem for six minutes, thus the name "66."

The leader sorts out and summarizes the small group discussions in front of a larger assembly of the groups of six. This has the advantage of a brainstorming session because it encourages a healthy competition between the groups. The leader plays an important role by collecting the best thinking from the group members before sharing it with the assembled group.

15. There are two methods associated with the *random word* technique. One is the organized method in which the group limits itself to a specific area of a problem for a specific amount of time. Following this time period, the group moves to another area of the problem and so on. Then, by reviewing the parts which were studied, usually new ideas or solutions are generated concerning the whole problem.

The second type is the free association method. Words are selected and connections are forced between them and the stated problem. This stimulates new combinations, intangible ideas, designs, etc, because the ideas feed upon each other and result in imaginative possibilities.

16. The *synectics technique* developed by W.J. Gordon uses analogies and metaphors to stretch the mind in new directions in order to increase idea output. The main thrust of this approach is to develop new perspectives in looking at and solving problems. The technique is dependent on the ability of the individual to "make the strange familiar" and "make the familiar strange."

In the first phase of this method, the person is asked to make a connection between something with which they are unfamiliar, and something with which they are familiar. For example, the unfamiliar blow hole of a whale can be associated with the escaping steam from an overheated automobile radiator. This connection leads to imagining a mechanism for the auto radiator which releases excessive pressure in the system.

In phase two, symbolic, personal, fantasy, and direct analogies are used to convert ideas of familiar, real items or situations into unfamiliar, unreal abstract items or situations. A steam-leaking automobile radiator may be thought of as a source of power if the escaping steam is harnessed to drive a paddle wheel on an air-conditioning unit. When members of the synectics group discuss these "strange," "far-out" ideas their interaction produces many new and "wilder" ideas. The analogies and metaphors used when trying to come up with ideas stimulate free-flow utilization of many areas of a person's experiences. Ideas can then be force-fit to generate potential problem solutions. The use of ideas generated from an individual's fantasy and personal experiences opens many doors which normally are kept closed by traditional, habitual, socially dictated thought patterns. When individuals are guided through the synectics process properly, each contributor becomes a veritable fountain of thoughts which, when joined with other fountains, produce rivers of invaluable, productive, imaginative ideas.

Direct analogies are connections made from the plant and animal world to the essence of the problem. The idea of using a caisson for underwater constructions came from the inspiration of a man watching the way a shipworm forms a tube for itself as it bores through wood.

Personal analogies are connections a person makes between himself/herself and some object, and the connections are expressed in terms of how it "feels" to be that thing. The person attempts to capture the essence of being the object.

Symbolic analogies are abstractions through the use of two conflicting words which are compressed to yield the "essence" of the situation. This is the most difficult of the analogies because the mind is forced to deal with totally abstract, conflicting ideas. This is sometimes called a "book title" and a "compressed conflict" in the synectics process.

Fantasy analogies are wishing, supposing, or imagining things with unlimited resources and imagination. Dream it, and it's possible.

All of these analogies use metaphors and similies to *stretch* the mind and *release* creative thoughts without concern or prejudgment.

The sequence of events in a synectics session is as follows:

Techniques and Strategies for Thinking Creatively

1. The problem-as-given (PAG) is stated to the group.

2. The purge. Participating members share possible solutions to the PAG. The purpose is to clear the mind and share thoughts on actual potential solutions. Following this stage, the participants are able, through analogies, to begin the thought processes and idea formation relative to the problem.

3. Now the problem is perceived in a different manner. This is called the Problem-as-understood (PAU).

4. With this new insight, the leader, through the use of evocative questioning, keeps the group's focus on its task.

The use of analogies and making the familiar strange adds new dimensions to the group's thought processes which can be applied to the problem. This transformation is the essence of creative thinking. Additional information on this method can be obtained from Synectics Education Systems, Cambridge, Massachusetts.

Creativity is an adventure, a journey into a life of greater personal reward and happiness. It is a philosophy based on the premise that whatever the mind can imagine the person can achieve. Each person is potentially creative. To have creativity and to exercise it takes courage. Courage to believe in one's self and courage to overcome obstacles generated by others. We all have the responsibility to recognize, stimulate, and utilize to its fullest the creativity within ourselves and those around us. The greater perceptual abilities of the creative person increases awareness and makes him/her a more effective change agent. The empathy, trust, and mutual respect this person exhibits toward self and peers are the seeds which, sown on fertile soil, blossom into the flowers of creativity.

The professional nurse has an obligation not only to demonstrate creative thought but also to bring it out in others. A creative mind not only develops the mental capacity of the individual but reduces the problems associated with stress in the body.

Creative leadership and teamwork are necessary to cope with our everchanging society. Now, more than ever, the talents of creative leaders are needed in the nursing profession. Support and encouragement of group members by leadership is essential when dealing with societal changes. The holistic approach of using both convergent and divergent thinking is resolving conflicts and in planning for the future should be used by all concerned persons.

The person who balances imaginative thought and reality is well on the way to becoming a self-actualized person. A commitment to thinking creatively is the highest compliment one can pay one's self. By making this commitment both to yourself and to others the world will become a better place; your innovative, creative, and imaginative way of life will cause it.

Chapter 6

Managing Creativity

There are four fundamentals in managing creativity: the leader must know and understand him/herself; know and understand other people; improve all forms of communication, eg, verbal, nonverbal, written, etc; and possess an in-depth knowledge of creativity and the creative process. It is the lack of these skills that cause managers to be ineffective as leaders. Leaders who are humanistic in their approach to members of their organization motivate others because they demonstrate that they care.

In order for creativity to exist in an organization, it is imperative that there be an environment to support creative human behavior. This is a major prerequisite to thinking and allowing creative thoughts to emerge. The first important factor should be an environment in which there is mutual trust between participants and leaders.

There are four specific goals that must be rigorously perceived by any organization bent on becoming more creative and adaptive to its rapidly changing environment.

1. It must reduce the amount of excessive structure to an absolute minimum.
2. It must increase the range of individual and organizational inputs.
3. It must introduce creative catalysts to spark the organization.
4. It must reward innovative behavior.[1]

The climate produced by these goals allows each person to contribute ideas and concepts without fear of intimidation. High trust levels exhibited by members of the group allow each person to bring forth ideas with a minimal risk to their ego. The change agent (manager) must develop a supportive environment. "Managers must take a close look at how they can open up their organizations, broaden the range and variety of information, increase organizational tolerance for diversity and complexity-staffing patterns as well as the organizational goals and activities."[1] Managing creativity is an ongoing dynamic program that allows people to use their minds to develop better ways of handling present and future problems. The freedom to express oneself is very important if the leader wants creative thinking to take place in the organization. The environment must be open so that individuals are allowed to think and share ideas without being ridiculed, either verbally or nonverbally, or held in high suspicion. The organizational climate must be conducive for self-expression. By building this trust environment, elements that impede or hinder creative thinking and creative problem solving will be minimized.

A creative environment will aid in the flow of ideas and increase the effectiveness of the organization, because more people participate in a positive manner. Exposure to this environment will enhance a person's ability to think in creative ways.

Organizations that are counterproductive in managing creativity seem to have an excessive need to control employee activities. These less creative organizations place an inordinately high value on organizational charts, manuals, job descriptions, budgets, and adherence to company policies. Hence, they recognize only one "correct" way to accomplish a task and overemphasize the factor of time.

Organizations that encourage creativity are usually characterized by the following:

1) Little formalization or standardization.
2) Performance based on ends versus means and have long time perspectives on accomplishing tasks.
3) Open communication network and channels.
4) Emphasis on tasks allowing intrinsic rewards to individuals.
5) Reduce the amount of structure to an absolute minimum.
6) Structure and clarity are needed at the goal level but not at the means level.
7) A high degree of participation and autonomy from all participants.
8) A high degree of job satisfaction.
9) Independence of judgment, allowing members to make decisions.
10) Worker preference for complexity.
11) Worker is objective in separating information from its source.
12) Relativistic, worker is familiar with overall production process.
13) Worker's sense of humor encouraged.
14) System allows employees to dream, contemplate, and realize their fantasies.
15) System recognizes and rewards creative activities and behavior patterns even though they do not conform to an expected pattern.
16) A positive attitude toward the capabilities of the worker is expressed by management.
17) Management and individuals know when to separate idea-finding from solution-finding.

18) Leaders manage indirectly by utilizing suggestions.

19) Managers promote worker self-esteem and pride.

20) Managers recognize where discipline should be asserted, and then assert it.

21) Managers have a high degree of respect and appreciation for creative talent.

22) Creative managers must sublimate their own egos.[2-5]

It is important to recognize that not all tasks or operations of an organization need to be creative all of the time. In many cases an attempt to utilize creative thinking where it may not be required or sought could hurt the effectiveness or productivity of the group. Problems which affect both the leader and the worker require an atmosphere in which all parties can participate in a constructive manner. Awareness of the kinds of environments that foster or smother creative thinking is the essence of managing creativity. Today's affluent society can be attributed to man's ability to produce new ideas through creativity. In fact, most of the great benefits that we have today have been produced or invented by people who are still living. The creative endeavors of these individuals have made it possible for us to enjoy the good health and prosperity which we value so highly. The need for more creative people in our society is even greater today. If our living standards and those of the rest of the world are to continue improving, more and more creative solutions will be required to solve our problems. If present and future problems are to be solved creatively, there is an urgent need to provide an environment that allows people to contribute their thoughts and express their creativity without condemnation.

When creativity and the creative process is recognized as an art with its own modus operandi, it can become a viable process which, if properly used, can help achieve the objectives and goals of an organization or group.

An organizational philosophy that stresses creativity as one of its goals and encourages it at all levels will increase the opportunities for its occurrence. It is important for an organization to recognize the qualities of the creative mind and to establish an environment in which the creative individual can flourish.

While it is important for an organization to be creative, it is equally important for the organization to recognize the characteristics of the creative individual.

The creative individual is:

- different from other people, and knows it;
- more independent than the average person;
- more interested in the problem, and it is the problem which proves to be the driving force;
- functioning best when deadlines are imposed;

- able to distinguish between the information and the source of the information;
- more impulse-ridden, more irrational, but still with superior controls;
- apparently wasting time when, in fact, he is allowing himself to be exposed to a wide range of stimuli so that he can get a grasp of the total situation;
- apt to work hard for long periods of time because he finds the problem challenging;
- future-oriented rather than past-reliant;
- open-minded and does not make snap judgments;
- a nonconformist in the area of generating ideas and sometimes not concerned about social norms;
- aggressive, self-assertive, and quick with suggestions;
- not bothered by working on problems which may not have clear-cut and unambiguous answers;
- apt to be flexible, and not a rigid follower of rules;
- happy toying with ideas and wants freedom to explore new ideas on his own;
- more impressed with what he doesn't know than what he does know;
- able to make distinctions in the grey area, rather than just black and white;
- thirsty for new and unusual experiences;
- able to take things lightly and with a sense of humor;
- endowed many times with above average intelligence;
- flexible and can accept change;
- intuitive;
- introverted;
- rejective of external constraints;
- highly self-confident;
- desirous of recognition and praise;
- able to make connections that may not be apparent to other people;
- goal-oriented, not method-oriented;
- competent, and possesses and employs different strategies and skills developed through the use of the imagination.

After reviewing the features of creative organizations and the traits of the creative individual, similarities between the two should be apparent. Both the creative organization and creative individuals must be present if the organization hopes to be creative in its endeavors. The "knowledge" explosion which seems to be intensifying in our society requires that both managers and individuals utilize their creative abilities.

The resources that are spent on our increasing technological development must be matched in the area of actualizing human potential. Man, by using his creative abilities, can make technology his servant rather than his master.

As stated earlier, one of the prime conditions for managing creativity is to provide a high trust environment. Employees must be able to freely express their ideas. It is important to recognize that different people express their ideas through different communication channels. The manager must be aware of these differences. In addition, he/she must be a good listener and must show sincere interest in the person's ideas. Sharing ideas and concerns by both managers and workers, without censure or rebuke, is an essential element in the management of creative environments.

In conjunction with the sharing of ideas, action taken on the submitted ideas should be fed back to the contributing individual or group. This action usually increases and stimulates more ideas from the contributing participants. This trust environment will encourage more creative thinking about organizational problems and insure that new or original ideas are never turned away without serious consideration. It is all right to have radical ideas as long as they are not detrimental to the organizational goals. Organizational training and encouragement by management assists individuals in thinking creatively about everything that is being done by the organization. Constructing this environment facilities the organization's goal and the individual's needs.

Any organization can be set up to encourage or to discourage creativity. A leader who plans to facilitate creativity will usually have a wide span of control as opposed to a narrow one. The person who is able to delegate authority and responsibility to others, and allow them to be relatively free in making their own decisions, encourages creativity rather than conformity. It is important to realize that, if an organization is to foster and maintain creativity, top management must set the climate for creativity in the organization. Support by management will enhance the creativity of the individual in the organization. The supportive environment and the recognition of individual creativity will permeate all levels of management. However, in addition to favorable attitudes or support by management, there also must be a responsive attitude from the worker toward the positive climate created by management. It is a two-way street. Neither the management nor the worker can operate in a vacuum.

It is difficult to describe all the attitudes and attributes of the creative manager. However, the following can serve as a guide for the manager in the development and maintenance of a working atmosphere which will foster creativity. A manager should be creative to inspire creativity. However, while the manager may not exhibit exceptional creative ability, the manager recognizes, encourages, and supports creativity in others. It is imperative that the manager possess an understanding of the creative process. Understanding some of the basic psychological characteristics of creativity, the things that block or discourage creativity, and different approaches used to enhance creativity are important concerns to the leader.

A creative manager sets the PACE: *Positive Attitude Changes Everything.* Also, he/she gives HOPE: *Honesty, Organizational skills, Positive thinking,* and a high degree of *Enthusiasm.* He/she is future-oriented because he realizes that he cannot change his yesterdays. By awakening, stimulating, activating, and enlarging the potential creativity of employees, the creative manager establishes his/her work unit as an effective, well-functioning production instrument that produces at optimum levels. He/she acts as a catalyst in developing and maintaining the creative environment and in recognizing employees as valuable problem-solving resources. His/her holistic and humanistic approach to both persons and processes within his jurisdiction acts to reduce costs, improve quality, and most important, ensure a creative working atmosphere which can be depended upon in future organizational plans.

The atmosphere generated for the workers by the managers and proper direction of the creative worker's ability ensures functional teamwork and coordinated activities among the workers in the unit. This work unit is flexible to process organizational and production demands yet highly sensitive to the human element.

The creative manager in discussions with employees tactfully nudges them in a chosen direction without disclosing his/her actual position. This management by ambiguity is an art-form that creative individuals can respond to with positive behavior. Approaching the individual in this fashion ensures the integrity of the worker's pride, self-esteem, and ensures self-direction. The manager's discerning manner in asking questions is highly effective and recognized by the workers. The manager's questions are usually probing, stimulating, provocative, and correctly timed to help the person develop innovative approaches to problem solving. This managerial strategy encourages a person's imagination in resolving conflicts. This communication exchange is very important and held in high regard by both parties. While definitely people-oriented, the manager will take the initiative when necessary to discipline a worker or to reconcile differences between workers. He/she is not afraid to act or assert himself if the need arises, all the while knowing that creative individuals are extremely sensitive to any actual or implied criticisms of their ideas.

While there is no one way to manage, the creative manager uses different management styles to respond to the variety of situations he may encounter in the performance of his duties. He/she is able to contain personal feelings when expectations are not met.

There is no such thing as a "perfect" manager, but the creative leader comes as close as possible to perfection because he/she wants to maximize the output of the creative persons within his domain. He/she is willing to accept and incorporate ideas from others which may be better than his own. He/she is a good loser as well as a good winner. He/she is a fair, competitive person and is able to control emotions even when they are provoked or tested.

A creative manager not only knows the way, but shows the way. He/she is sincere and has faith in the creative process because his belief is in people rather than budgets, buildings, and other material items. The manager is optimistic in his/her attitude toward solving problems. By this optimistic attitude he/she instills and encourages self-confidence in others. Deferment of judgment is maintained throughout the project. A balance is kept between his/her emotions and external influences relative to the position. This emotional stability is a positive characteristic that others are eager to follow, but are not compelled to obey.

The creative leader is an effective decision-maker and recognizes that making decisions is a fundamental management responsibility. While decision making involves risk, the decisions must be made in the present even though the result may affect future organizational plans. When it is necessary to make tough value judgments, he/she demonstrates tack and diplomacy with all parties concerned.

Although changes are frequent and difficult to predict, the creative manager is an effective planner. He/she is able to shape future events rather than simply predict them. Prediction is a passive and ineffective management tool.

In managing creativity, the creative leader sets deadlines for the tasks to be completed. Deadlines help motivate creative people to overcome the inertia that besets them when assigned new tasks. Joint agreement on a time frame helps the creative individual sense the significance of the project and gain added personal recognition.

When assigning tasks to a creative individual, it is essential that the manager explain the need, importance, and constraints of the project. Once the creative individual understands the problem and its parameters, it is best to leave him/her alone to use imagination and ingenuity. Poor initial managerial guidance can result in large amounts of wasteful thinking. Many creative individuals have a narrow area of interest. The worker believes that only he/she is capable of creating a solution and this belief reinforces his self-image and ego.

The creative individual attaches a high value to personal recognition, prestige, reward, feedback, etc, from his/her immediate manager. These intrinsic rewards have a much higher priority than the extrinsic values of salary and promotion.

Another managerial responsibility is to provide training for creativity. A leader allows and encourages people to attend classes and formal training programs which enhance their ability to understand and internalize creative thinking. This behavior on the part of the manager indicates to the worker that the management strongly supports the implementations of creative thought processes and behaviors of the individual. The implementation of training sessions allows the individual a period of adjustment while his/her work environment is gearing up to a more creative climate. The effective training program should be followed up by the manager to ensure that the employees are applying the information and techniques which they learned. If the manager constantly monitors post-training session activities, then he promotes and encourages employee initiative, resourcefulness, and creativity. He/she accomplishes this through both formal and informal channels of communication.

To further develop and enhance creative thinking the organization has a "quiet room" that is accessible to all workers. This room includes inspiring and stimulating resources for mental excursions. These mental excursions can lead to new, original, and important breakthroughs. The environment of this room includes works of art, music (individual headsets), comfortable seating arrangements, walls or boards for writing, posting and cataloging ideas which encourage reflection and incubation of ideas relative to an assigned task. The decor includes a large carpeted open area for meditation and physical relaxation. Refreshments conducive to the encouragement of creative thought can reduce the mental fatigue associated with the process of generating ideas. These refreshments can be juices, nuts, fruit, or other high energy foods. This "think-tank" room allows the creative individual the freedom to be more productive during the initial stage of engaging in the problem. Adjacent to this area a library which contains books, periodicals, and audio and video tapes can be used as additional sources of reference and inspiration.

It cannot be overemphasized that the creative person is the heart of the organization. He is continuously conceiving new and better ways of doing things, devising money-saving methods, suggesting means of increasing productivity, thinking of new product ideas, and offering ideas for increasing sales and profits.

Five "A's" which are important to the leader who manages creative employees are: Attention, Appreciation, Articulation, Awareness and Admiration.

First, *attention* is paid to the worker by actively listening to his/her needs and concerns. Second, *appreciation* is given for all contributions made by the worker. Third, *articulation* of all directions, instructions, and communications so the worker readily understands what is expected. Fourth, there is an *awareness* that the "whole" individual is of paramount importance to the realization of the organizational goals and objectives. Fifth, *admiration* is freely expressed to acknowledge that a person's work is worthwhile and respected. Incorporating these five A's into the managerial functions provides recognition, prestige, gratification, and feedback that motivate creative individuals to maintain their pride and continue their high value of self-worth in the organization. Creative people like to feel that their particular talent or ability is acknowledged.

While it is important for the manager to recognize and appreciate individual creative efforts, it is equally important to realize the effect of the interaction of individuals in a group setting. To heighten creative efforts on a given task it is sometimes best to expose a person to others not directly involved in the same task assignment. This exposure to others increases the data bank available to the individual. The ideas generated by others may trigger new ideas or may stimulate thoughts not previously generated. While some people may label these "bull sessions," they are not a waste of the company's time or money because the payoff in ideas is great.

At times a creative person needs to interact with other creative people in order to replenish and rejuvenate not only his/her information bank but also his/her social acceptance and self-assigned rewards. This sharing of ideas and listening to others for feedback helps the creative mind make new connections and reinforces the person's self-image. In group activities it is important to recognize that although the participants may appear to be either idle or unproductive, this seemingly unproductive time must be allowed by management because it is during this "idle" time that incubation is taking place. Many of the best ideas occur either during these times or immediately following periods of high concentration. An effective problem-solving group can, by mutual support, in a few hours produce what might take weeks or even months for a single individual to produce. This mutual support also facilitates greater risk taking by the individual members than if they were working alone. This is a by-product of the trust environment of the creative group. Also, the group allows great diversity and flexibility in approaches and strategies which change the direction of the problem-solution path. It takes time for the bud of an idea to blossom. While idle time may sometimes be unproductive, it is good to give individuals time off; this might be what is needed to start the creative juices flowing again. It is during the extended incubation period while a person is not directly involved in a task that the subconscious mind is able to bring to the foreground good ideas for the task solution. This is the "eureka" or "aha!" stage in creative thinking.

Managers must be aware of the quirks and foibles of creative individuals and groups. Creative people are nonconformists in the area of ideas and sometimes in the area of behavior. Understanding the idiosyncrasies of creative people, a wise manager will tolerate unconventional behavior because it is not actually harmful to the organization. However, the creative person seeks frequent evaluation from his/her immediate supervisor because he likes to know where he stands at all times. This compulsion for feedback is an essential motivational factor for creative individuals and groups.

Creative persons or groups should be assigned tasks which genuinely need their abilities. If they are given tasks which do not utilize their talents to the fullest, their thinking reverts to traditional processes. Their effectiveness as productive idea-generating entities is sharply reduced. Matching noncreative tasks with those who like them, and matching tasks which need creative thinking with creative individuals is one of the most neglected functions of management.

Creative managers can be stifled in their jobs because of company policies and procedure manuals. Although certain policies and procedures are necessary in an organization, the blind adherence to them can sometimes cause problems if a manager wishes to develop and encourage creativity on the job.

As a leader of creative people it is essential to be aware of the following considerations:

1. Keep your ego out of the way of your managing.

2. Try to keep calm and in control of a given situation. The people you manage will tend to act the same way.

3. Have a deep respect for the talents of creative people. Place a high value on creative thinking and innovation.

4. Have a high trust in your people.

5. Try to keep creative people happy even while realizing that they can be moody at times.

6. Allow creative people to experiment and try out their new ideas and thoughts. Allow them to change their minds or directions when working on a task. Allow flexibility.

7. Let creative people express themselves but do not take their expressions personally. Give the people as much latitude as is reasonable within the organization's policies.

8. Make suggestions in such a way that the creative person can accept them. Let the person feel that he/she is making the change and then thank the person for his/her good thinking. This positive attitude and behavior on the manager's part will give recognition to the person when needed. By managing indirectly, the manager places emphasis on

the creative individual's imagination and self-direction and effectively plays down his/her managerial role.

9. It is important for both parties to know their roles. The leader should know when discipline is needed and assert it. In this manner, the creative talent is guided in the tasks of the organization. Most people like to do a good job and the creative leader provides the incentive and opportunity for them to do it.

10. The creative leader uses the positive approach in accomplishing the organization's goals. It is this type of leadership that triggers the motivational force in creative people. A creative leader leads rather than pushes the group. Positive attitudes by the leader will motivate others to perform their tasks willingly and with interest and enthusiasm.

11. Creativity has its own rewards.

12. The creative manager is employee-centered. The leader makes his/her people feel important because he knows they are important to his career. The leader's results are usually measured by the results of the people within his area. Sometimes leaders forget this important fact, and many problems that arise are due to this lack of employee recognition.

13. The creative leader cares about the worker. People who manage others show that they care and their concern is expressed in their attitude and behavior.

14. The creative leader knows his workers. He/she assigns tasks that fit the person's abilities, and he also provides periodic feedback on the results of their efforts.

15. The manager's planning responsibilities are made easier because he/she allows self-direction among the workers.

16. The creative leader sets goals which are a great challenge both to himself/herself and to his workers but are achievable through creative thinking. The best can always be improved upon.

Our challenge, as creative individuals and managers, is to see that the people within an organization are able to cope with change in an effective and positive manner. This utilization of human resources helps both those in leadership positions and those in employee roles to function creatively in an ever-changing society.

Chapter 7

Five Step Creative Problem-Solving Process

The five step creative problem-solving process is attributed to Osborn[1] and refined by Parnes, Noller, and Biondi.[2] The five step process includes: fact-finding, problem-finding, idea-finding, solution-finding, acceptance-finding. A synopsis of each step of the process follows.

The *fact-finding step* attempts to identify all the facts related to the problem. The facts are gathered from personal experience, literature, other persons, records, and so forth. If the problem relates to a situation, the remarkable words: who, what, why, when, and how are used to trigger facts related to the problem. When the problem involves an object, words such as function, odor, sound, taste, color, and shape are useful in generating facts.

In the *problem-finding stage* the participant is involved in sensing problems or challenges for creative intervention. A list of stimulator words helps the participant to generate problem areas for consideration. The list includes common words that are capable of drawing associations in the participant's mind. For instance the words school? or work? or misunderstandings? are common words that are likely to bring problems to the participant's awareness. There are times when the participants come to a problem-solving session fully armed with problems to discuss. At other times, it may be necessary to have these lists of common words expressed as questions to stimulate their thinking. The statement of a problem for creative resolution is important. The creative problem is stated in the following way: "In what ways might I?" or "How might I?" Stating the problem in this way is likely to make problems seem amenable to resolution. It places a positive tone on the problem-solving situation and removes some of the negative attitudes associated with problems and their resolution. It is important to note that very often a problem turns out to be not one but many problems when it is stated in this way. Therefore, the subproblems are usually prioritized for consideration.

In the *idea-finding step* the SCAMPER (Eberle[3]) or similar format is used to purge the mind. SCAMPER stands for substitute, combine, adapt, modify, put to other uses, eliminate, and rearrange. The participant is encouraged to take ideas and use these words to help to change the idea. For instance, if the list of facts contained the words comb and brush, these two words are combined to be a combination one piece article with a comb on one side and a brush on the other side. In this step the facts are expanded by the use of creative ideas. Or stated another way, observations or facts are manipulated by ideas.

Evaluation of the ideas takes place during the *solution-finding stage*. It is during this stage that the unusual ideas are critiqued for potential usefulness. It is acceptable to modify the ideas to improve their usefulness based on the criteria selected to judge the ideas. Criteria frequently used to judge ideas include the following: cost, moral or legal implications, timeliness, feasibility, effects on others, and so forth. The evaluation attempts to determine the best ideas to be used at the present time, retained for later use, or dropped from consideration.

Acceptance-finding relates to the implementation of the chosen strategie(s). Deliberate attempts are planned for gaining acceptance for the idea(s) before approaching the decision-makers with the solution. The question which permeates this stage is, "How might I gain acceptance for this idea?" In this stage, it is well to consider who else might be helpful in getting the idea across as well as who will be affected by the idea. It is appropriate to ask, "What is the worst thing that can happen to the idea?" and then to try to think of ways to overcome the potential obstacles. A definitive timetable is established for implementing each stage of the idea so that the idea is not put away or lost.

The five step creative problem-solving process is facilitated by utilizing the principles of deferred judgment, brainstorming, and incubation. *Deferred judgment* is the act of deferring evaluation until after all the ideas are out on the table. Premature evaluation of ideas results in limiting the possibility for all the ideas to emerge. Deferring judgment allows the participants to generate ideas in a freewheeling manner. No idea is considered good, bad, or indifferent during the freewheeling stages of the problem-solving process. The stages which allow judgment are the solution-finding and the acceptance-finding stages. It takes time for participants to learn to defer judgment. Exercises can be helpful in producing this behavior. Simply introduce the participants to the principle of deferred judgment and then have them generate ideas without judging them. Each time a participant says, "It won't work, we tried it before" or "They won't let us do that," the leader interjects a reminder regarding deferred judgment. It is important to point out that chuckles, snickers, frowns, smiles, and so forth are also judgment behaviors; therefore, they are discouraged just like verbal judgments.

Brainstorming is a technique for generating large numbers of ideas. During the brainstorming process, deferred judgement is essential. Brainstorming allows for all the participants to be involved in idea generation, simultaneously. A time frame is established, usually ten to twenty minutes. Then the participants are encouraged to give their ideas verbally and a recorder records the responses. If the brainstorming process slows down, the leader can stimulate the participants to think further by asking for ten more ideas or throwing out the words magnify, minify, put to other uses, and so forth. The participants tend to help one another think by spurring ideas that arise from each other's contributions. This situation is referred to as hitchhiking on someone else's idea to produce another idea. Ideas generated through brainstorming range from far-out ideas to traditional ideas. The process is focused on the quantity rather than the quality of the ideas.

Closely associated with the principles of deferred judgment and brainstorming is the principle of *incubation*. All of the ideas that come from the brainstorming session have the ability to gain in usability after a period of time elapses and more thinking ensues in relation to the ideas. Putting ideas away for a period of time and then bringing them out again allows the participant time to generate additional ideas and to modify or expand the original ideas. This process is called incubation.

The creative problem-solving process, including deferred judgment, brainstorming, and incubation, is a powerful tool for resolving challenges which confront society. The process is fun as well as encompassing for the participants. Each step of the process can be filled with exercises that help to stimulate creativity of the participants. Many of these exercises are included throughout this volume. Most importantly, the steps of the process do not have rigid boundaries between them. If the participants get to the solution-finding step and need more facts, it is essential that fact-finding be done again. This flexibility between the steps allows for generation of useful ideas to emerge and for problems to be thoroughly assessed before solutions are determined and implemented.

The essential ingredients for creative problem solving include: problems, interested persons, environments that encourage free thinking and risk-taking, and time. The goals of creative problem solving is to find answers that have utility and perhaps novelty for meeting challenges and bringing them to a successful conclusion. Examples of problems that are attacked using the five-step process appear in Chapters 10 and 11.

Divergent-Convergent Thinking

The five step creative problem-solving process deliberately forces the participant to use a combination of convergent and divergent thinking.

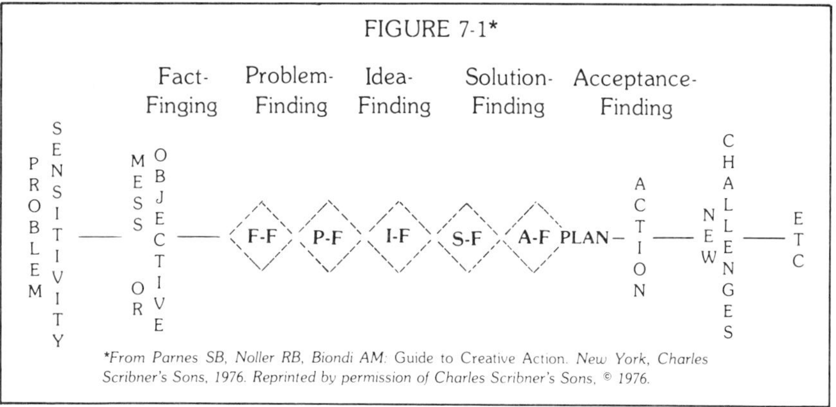

*From Parnes SB, Noller RB, Biondi AM: Guide to Creative Action. New York, Charles Scribner's Sons, 1976. Reprinted by permission of Charles Scribner's Sons. © 1976.

Convergent thinking is narrowing down an idea—fine tuning it—while divergent thinking expands thinking—opens it up. Convergent thinking is closely associated with the researchers attempts to narrow down the problem, cutting out the extraneous variables and sharply focusing on the key issue to be investigated. Divergent thinking is open, free, and takes in just as much as possible. Divergent thinking allows one to go off on tangents and excursions in order to gain the broadest perspective of the problem that is possible. Using a combination of convergent and divergent thinking allows the participant the freedom to explore in a freewheeling fashion before zeroing in on the major components of a problem. The participant is encouraged to move from convergent thinking back to divergent thinking and vice versa at periodic intervals during the problem-solving process. The tired feeling that frequently is associated with convergent thinking as the problem is narrowed to minute proportions is counteracted by the light, free, unrestrained feeling associated with divergent thinking. Divergent thinking is somewhat like a child skipping merrily through a field of wild flowers, changing direction at will, bending to sniff the fragrance, exploring the swaying faces, snipping an occasional bud, delighting in a busy bee, and so forth. As the child takes each opportunity to explore the environment, change direction at will, and go on unscheduled excursions, so too can the creative problem solver. Many of the usual constraints imposed on individuals involved in solving problems are purposefully removed to let in new air and remove the cobwebs which interfere with producing refreshing new ideas.

Figure 7-1 is a graphic illustration of the creative problem-solving steps using convergent and divergent thinking.

Defining the Problem

The resolution of problems seldom starts with a well defined problem.

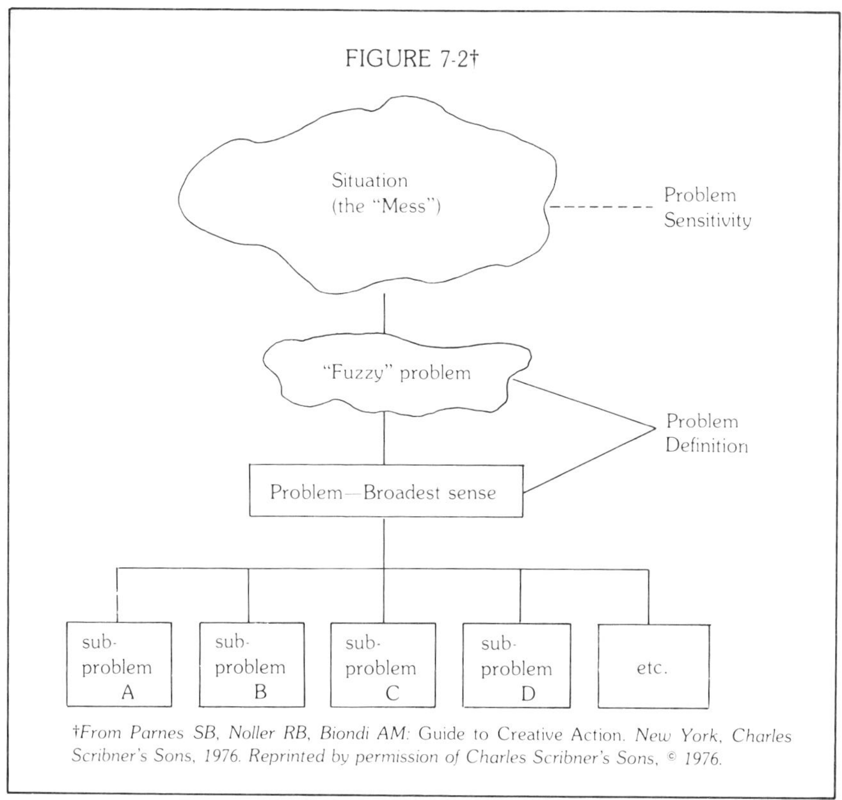

†From Parnes SB, Noller RB, Biondi AM: Guide to Creative Action. New York, Charles Scribner's Sons, 1976. Reprinted by permission of Charles Scribner's Sons, © 1976.

More often the problem is poorly defined, and this makes it difficult to know how to use our problem-solving ability to effectively resolve the problem. Figure 7-2 is an illustration of the situation at this point in the early resolution of problems. The situation begins with a mess. Then the problem is defined by identifying "fuzzy problems" associated with the "mess." The fuzzy problems are converted into broad problem statements which usually result in a group of subproblems.

Stating the problem adequately is a vital step in the creative problem-solving process. You have come a long way when the fuzzy problem and mess are sorted out. As most situations are infiltrated with messes and fuzzy problems, the participant learns to enjoy the challenge of delving into the mess and making it better. The participant, who does not work on the solution to the problem, becomes part of the problem. Sensing problems, being involved in resolving them, and helping others to be involved is a challenge open to all participants.

Child's Creativity—Adult Problem Solving

The ability to use the creative problem solving successfully is closely associated with the participants willingness to recapture the free spirit and intellectual curiosity of the child. The child goes merrily about the world asking questions that seem to have no ready answers, but this does not interfere with the child's intense interest in solving problems and understanding his/her world. The child may get frustrated at the lack of answers to his/her questions but the determination to find answers keeps the child's problem-solving ability alive. The child uses the frustration created by a confusing situation to come up with novel ideas for solving problems—ones that are frequently rejected by the adults that are overwhelmed by his/her ability to get around the roadblocks that interfere with the child's desires or wishes. The child has an enthusiasm for participating in problem resolution. This enthusiasm is partly responsible for the success associated with the immature problem-solving skills that the child possesses. The child explores the world with the freshness of a spring day after a gentle rain. Adults need to copy the child's spirit of inquiry and sense the value of approaching problem situations from a positive frame of reference. The child enjoys problem solving; adults can, too.

I'm reminded of the little girl whose mother sent her to the store for a loaf of bread. She left the house and turned in the wrong direction. Not finding the store she returned and told her mother, "They tore the store down!" The child's simplistic approach to problem solving did not interfere with her ability to find new answers. She found this unlikely solution a perfectly acceptable alternative. Her naivity was refreshing and brought humor into the situation. She made a mistake but she was not caught without a potential solution to the problem she faced. She thought the situation through, used her limited repetoire of past experiences, and generated an alternative that made the solution seem plausible to her. Obviously, the child's mother was not pleased with the child's efforts at problem solving no matter how diligently the child worked to come up with the explanation. However, this innovative child's explanation is superior to the adult's explanations that the problem cannot be solved. Both the child and adult have problems to address: to the child everything is possible, to the adult little is possible. Both ends of the spectrum need to be tempered to produce ideas that are viable and acceptable for problem resolution.

Part II

Nursing Applications

Introduction

An attempt is made, in this section, to focus on ways to stimulate the creative potential of nurses in role-specific situations. The roles, selected for inclusion in the discussion, are person, faculty facilitator, student, and manager. Although special attention is paid to a selected role in a specific chapter, it is possible to modify information in other chapters to use with more than one role. Therefore, the chapters should not be viewed as discrete entities, but as being interrelated with each other.

One chapter is devoted to nurturing the creative potential of clients. Again, this chapter is not meant to stand alone. Many ideas found in other chapters are equally relevant to the client as well as to the nurse.

The discussion of the nurse as a person is based on psychological, philosophical, and theological imperatives. If at times, the message sounds evangelical, we must apologize in advance. Our belief is that the nurse, as a person, is a key element which influences success or failure as a professional helper. Our message is not meant to be a directive. Rather, it is meant to be self-stimulating. Whatever the consequences, our beliefs that the self as person plays a significant part in each practicing nurse's approach to the client is clearly documented in the upcoming discussion. We hope that our ideas, drawn from a variety of sources, will stimulate your thinking and warrant your consideration of an intensive exploration of this aspect of the preparation and maturation of the professional nurse.

The framework proposed for generating creative potential is based on the background material presented in the first part of the book. The framework consists of four components: the five-step creative problem-solving process, increasing perceptual awareness, use of all the senses, and fostering activity of the right and left hemisphere of the brain.

Exercises are presented to increase creativity. These exercises attempt to stimulate thinking in new ways by decreasing the use of habit, making unusual associations between ideas, making new connections between ideas, using the imagination, and using the process of deferred judgment and incubation in problem situations. The exercises can be modified and used in a variety of situations. Research supports that creativity is nurtured through the use of these exercises. The exercises can be fun. The major intent of the exercises is to increase the use of the right hemisphere of the brain which is responsible for creative thinking.

References are cited, throughout the section, to introduce experts who facilitate understanding of creativity. The reader is encouraged to pursue the original works to gain a greater appreciation of the intent of these authors. In addition, the reference list at the end of the book offers many opportunities for expanding awareness of creativity and its use in the problem-solving process.

There is a disproportionately large number of women in the nursing profession. At times, this factor can be an asset. When discussing creativity, this situation is a plus factor as studies show that women are more creative than men. How then can we manipulate this advantage to make the nursing profession benefit? The proposed answer to this question sounds quite simple but is actually quite complex. We need to help nurses express the creative potential they possess. Implementation of this idea can only be successful if attention is paid to numerous variables which impact on the nursing situation and profession. What are some of the variables which influence the creative posture of the nursing profession? The following list is representative but not exhaustive:

1) Nurses must value creativity as important to the profession.
2) Environments where nurses perform must allow the freedom necessary for creativity to emerge.
3) Rewards for performance must reflect an awareness of the value of creative pursuits.
4) Educational programs for preparing nurses must allow opportunities for developing creative potential.
5) A reawakening and emphasis on the humane aspects of nursing are essential.
6) Client-centered nursing practice must continue to replace functional structured nursing practice.
7) Flexibility in thought and action must be the building blocks for the profession.
8) Autocratic climates must be replaced with democratic climates.
9) Nurses must be supportive of one another's achievements in order to stimulate continual creative activities.
10) Nurses must possess the self-confidence to become risk-takers.
11) Nurses must have a personal as well as a professional commitment to the advancement of the profession.

Chapter 8

Creativity and Creative Persons

All great ideas are controversial. Or have been controversial at one time.

George Seldes

There is a lot more information known today about creativity than there was in past years. Still, the knowledge in the area is incomplete, and some authorities disagree with other authorities about creativity and how to nurture it. The increased attention that is being given to understanding creativity and creative persons is an indication that significant numbers of people are genuinely interested in the use of creativity for helping to solve problems of every magnitude. Additionally, as a wide range of disciplines are already interested in creativity and unleashing creative potential in their members, it is evident that creativity is valued even when it is not completely understood.

It is interesting that so much can be stated about creativity while concurrently so much remains to be learned about it. To date, the tip of the iceberg is all that has been explored. In addition, there is not a great deal that is predictable about creativity. Perhaps that is one of the things that makes creativity exciting to consider. There is still an elusive nature about creativity that makes it both easy and hard to understand, at exactly the same time.

Maslow[1] suggests that the human being has naturalistic tendencies which are capable of molding him/her into humaneness. Among those tendencies are creativity, spontaneity, authenticity, caring for others, capacity for loving, and the yearing for truth. He calls these tendencies *embryonic potentialities*. If Maslow's assumptions are correct, it is important that emphasis be placed on structuring the environment so that these embryonic tendencies in individuals are developed to the fullest extent. The tendencies that Maslow identifies are essential to professionals who interact with other human beings in a helping way. The effective interactions of significant persons result in a climate which permits, fosters, helps, or encourages the embryonic-tendencies, described above, to become actualized. When these tendencies are supported and nurtured the end result is self-knowing and self-acceptance. Self-knowledge is an established vehicle for self-improvement; however, it is not the only way to achieve this goal. Self-knowledge and self-improvement are valuable ends but they are not achieved without a struggle.

Zinker[2] proposes that creativity is the expression of the full range of personal experiences and sense of uniqueness with others. He suggests that creativity is a brave act because the person asserts a willingness to risk failures and criticism in order to witness a new and refreshing existence.

Martindale[3] notes that creative people process information differently. For instance, when given a new solution to a problem, creative people tend to offer additional ideas and solutions while overlooking or ignoring the defects and problems with the suggested plan of action. Less creative people find fault with the solution, focus on the defects, and lose sight of exploring the potential outcomes of the solution or ideas that are presented. This difference in the way creative people process information is significant as creative persons continue forward movement during problem solving while less creative persons engage in backward movement.

As Martingale[3] suggests, creative persons, when confronted with novelty, get excited and involved, while less creative persons turn suspicious and even hostile. Novelty is fun for the person who is creatively inclined. It provides a stimulus for ideation which is valued by creative persons but has less value for their less creative counterparts.

Moustakas[4] indicates that a creative person is not tied to the past, present, or future. He/she lives to respond to each situation from a somewhat neutral position of "openness." Each situation is viewed from this open stance allowing the use of all his/her personal resources to respond to the situation as it unfolds. These encounters with life allow the participant to relate to the demands made by existence in new and challenging ways.

In Martindale's[3] research, he found that creativity is not derived from being curious about the surroundings but by combining curiosity with the effective use of right brain wave activity. He ties creativity to physiological function of the brain suggesting that creative persons produce less alpha frequencies when they are relaxing and produce more alpha frequencies when they are working on an imaginative problem. There is, however, still a great deal of controversy regarding the differences in brain activity associated with creative or less creative persons.

An exceptional quality of creativity is that it is cumulative. Persons who feel the satisfaction generated from creative expression have the desire to continue to create. Therefore, one creative act tends to encourage another creative act. Creative acts produce positive feelings which trigger the participant's desire to have the feelings rekindled and rekindled. Through this process, creativity becomes a self-perpetuating act.

The use of creativity is intimately involved with the process of problem solving. Deliberate opportunities need to be provided for persons to use and develop their creative ability to be certain that creativity is expressed. It is no longer sensible to allow the expression of creativity to chance. Contributions to society from creative action are too valuable to be approached in this way.

Creativity—A Definition?

It does not seem appropriate to present one definition of creativity. Therefore, a definition is deliberately omitted from this volume. As a general guideline or framework, however, creativity is considered to be the ability to see problems in a different way and to generate new or significant solutions for resolving problems. The generation of ideas does not have to result in spectacular outcomes, but the idea-generating process has the potential to stimulate new insights that are useful.

Nurturing Creative Behavior

The assumption is made that nurses and nursing would benefit by nurturing creativity in the membership. Each of the nursing roles presented in this section have multifaceted tasks and responsibilities associated with the role. It is impossible to include an in-depth discussion of each of these tasks and responsibilities in this volume. Instead a sampling of the responsibilities related to the selected roles is used to illustrate how creativity and the process of creative problem solving can be nurtured in persons who assume each of the selected roles.

One caution is necessary when introducing the concept of creativity to persons who function mostly in the logical domain when solving problems. The language of creativity is certain to be confusing. These persons are not comfortable or accustomed to letting their minds flow freely, using their imaginations, daydreaming, and fantasizing. Persons steeped in logical reasoning sometimes discredit and ridicule the creative reasoning mode of thinking. It will take longer for persons who favor logical thinking to gain trust in the creative problem-solving process and to allow themselves the opportunity to explore their creative thinking capacity. Some persons are not able to break away from or vary their cherished logical way of thinking to try their creative capabilities. While these persons may lose personally from this stance, a more serious situation is the possibility that they will stifle the interest of their colleagues who desire the opportunity to think creatively.

> *Less than fifteen per cent of the people do any original thinking on any subject....The greatest torture in the world for most people is to think.*
>
> Luther Burbank

No problem is too small or insignificant to warrant the use of creativity in its resolution. Every problem situation deserves to be approached through a combination of creative and logical thinking. If this stance is assumed, the door is kept open for unusual and innovative ideas to emerge from all problem situations. The combined approach to problem solving has the potential to result in spectacular achievements during problem resolution. In solving problems creatively, it is equally important not to rule out the obvious. Many times the obvious is ruled out and the best solution to the problem is unintentionally overlooked.

Many questions still remain to be answered regarding the preparation of health professionals and the most effective way to deliver health care services. While these questions remain unanswered it provides a golden opportunity to experiment with preparing professionals and delivering services in a variety of ways. Health professions must become aware of their creative abilities and be rewarded for using creativity. The greatest reservior of ideas for solving problems in the area of health lies dormant between the ears of health professionals and consumers, waiting to be discovered, expressed, and used effectively. The knowledge held by consumers and providers that is attainable for solving health problems is so great that it is difficult to imagine. Unlocking the human potential possessed by these two groups—providers and consumers—offers an opportunity to generate viable alternatives that can be effective for meeting the challenges posed by the current health care industry.

> *Every man is a consumer and ought to be a producer.*
> Ralph Waldo Emerson

Nurses, as the largest group in the health delivery service, hold a trump card for having opportunities to provide creative services which foster high level wellness. By virtue of the time nurses spend with clients, they have a unique opportunity to determine what care is delivered and to influence the expression of creativity in the clients they serve. The potentially powerful position that nurses can assume in the delivery of health care puts added responsibility on the members of the nursing profession to contribute positively to the improvement of health care services. The use of creativity in planning and implementing nursing care is a vehicle for reaching this goal. The time has long passed for nurses to be satisfied to function as handmaidens of the physician. In order for nurses to be viable in the big business arena of health care, independent thinking and action are essential.

Nursing is clearly an *art* and a *science*. The systematic creative problem-solving process is vital to the art of nursing while the research process is vital to the science of nursing. The combination of knowledges generated through creative problem solving and research holds the potential for propelling nursing to the forefront in the delivery of health care services. It is imperative to focus on ways to encourage creativity in nurses and nursing to be certain that the art of nursing is advanced at the same time that the science of nursing is receiving increased emphasis. If fact, one authority, DiCyan,[5] suggests that there is evidence to support that, by its very nature, science is antithetical to creativity. When the person elects the logical approach to problem solving, he/she is forced to ignore intuition which plays a major role in creativity. Consequently, it is necessary for the nursing profession to be aware that both science and creativity are vital for advancing the profession. Scientific methodologies in nursing are receiving increased attention, and it is now timely to concentrate effort on increasing the creative potential of members of the nursing profession.

> *Conventional people are roused to fury by departure from convention, largely because they regard such departure as a criticism of themselves.*
>
> Lord Russell

Nursing is a profession in transition. During this period, there are many opportunities to structure actions to capitalize on a variety of ways to foster the highest level of competence in nursing practitioners. The profession, individual nurses, consumers, and health care colleagues will all benefit from the efforts expended on these activities.

Chapter 9

Nurturing Creativity in the Nurse as a Person

It is essential to begin the discussion by focusing first on the nurse as a person. The person of a nurse is the primary therapeutic "instrument" of nursing. As such, the importance of the person of nurse cannot be underestimated. The nurse cannot be relegated to the position of being an extension of the technological and scientific advances associated with nursing and other health care professions. Rather, the nurse as a person must be a freely interacting human being who brings to the nursing profession a free and creative spirit of the mind. The nurse needs to understand self and the ramifications that self has on professional interactions. Inherent in the understanding of self is an examination of values, personal needs, interaction styles with others, patterns of coping with life stresses, and a willingness to change when change is warranted.

There are a variety of ways that the nurse as person can achieve these goals: conscious introspection, counseling, group discussion with colleagues or supervisors, personality testing, viewing interactions on videotapes, listening to audiotapes of verbal interactions, asking clients for evaluation, values clarification, and examining past and present actions.

Values Clarification

The values clarification process allows the nurse as a person to examine the values that influence the way he/she responds to situations and raises the level of consciousness associated with the decision-making process. The creative person often is in the forefront in changing traditional societal values. Creative persons are likely to change the way that reality is defined by focusing attention and change on traditional reinforcers. The early attention to value change makes the creative person at odds with the standards espoused by peers. This position places the creative person in a comfortless position. The knowledge of the eventual satisfaction that is associated with value change must sustain the creative person during the interim period. However, the creative person who risks changing values is prone to exclusion by peers, authorities, and family. It is clear that the creative person can cause discomfort in others due to their value preferences. Awareness of this risk helps the creative person to decide if the risks are worth the emotional investment.

Personal Needs

Examining personal needs is vital to self-understanding. The nurse as a person has needs that require attention in much the same way that the client's needs require attention. If the nurse as person is too engrossed in fulfilling personal needs, the possibility that the client's needs can be successfully met as well is decreased. The understanding that the personal needs drain the energy of the nurse as person is an essential concept to keep in mind as the nurse attempts to effectively use self as a therapeutic agent.

Interaction Styles

Interaction styles with individuals and groups are examined in an attempt to become aware of the positive and negative aspects of these interactions. It is not always possible to clearly and accurately perceive how one interacts with others. Verbal and nonverbal behaviors are explored and analyzed to develop accurate perceptions about the self that are likely to influence the nurse in professional transactions with clients, with colleagues, and with families of clients.

Coping Strategies

The nurse as a person has a repertoire of experiences which highlight how he/she copes with stressful life circumstances. Assessing these experiences helps to facilitate understanding of the way that coping occurs. The ability to cope successfully is paramount as the nursing role commonly occurs in stressful situations. The nurse as person who copes successfully is likely to be able to handle the stressful atmosphere where nursing frequently takes place and help clients to handle stress as well. The nurse as person who manages stress with difficulty is likely to negatively influence the behaviors of clients in stressful situations.

Change

The willingness to change when change is warranted emerges as a positive factor when discussing the nurse as person. If this posture is not assumed, the growth of the person is likely to be slowed significantly. This characteristic of the nurse as person is aimed at continually improving the personal attributes associated with the person who assumes the responsibility and obligations associated with a helping profession.

Self-appraisal

Self-appraisal is an essential component of self-understanding. In order for growth to take place, the nurse as person needs to consciously assess his/her behavior and determine if the behavior reflects a commitment to the nursing profession and to the clients that are served. In addition, the behaviors should reflect an emotionally satisfying personal life which is "becoming" towards the goal of self-actualization.

Creating Person

A primary goal of the individual is to create himself/herself. The newborn infant, no matter how miraculous he/she appears, is still an incomplete self. The immediate need of the newborn is to gain an understanding of the environmental and hereditory factors at his/her disposal and begin to create a person capable of surviving and flourishing in the world. The creation of a self takes on increasing importance as the child grows and is responsible for participating in society. The person who elects the profession of nursing joins the ranks of persons who prefers the opportunity to assist others.

The person assumes responsibility for creating a self that is able to see the needs of clients and to offer support during times of stress. The act of creation of helpers is not a simple process of molding volunteers to respond in a circumscribed format. Helpers come in many sizes, shapes, colors, intellects, religious persuasions, cultural backgrounds, and so forth. The creation of helpers from such diversified raw ingredients makes it imperative that the person seeking to be a helper assume the primary and major responsibility for creating a self as person that is eager to be part of a societal role that is given acclaim by the public because of the importance of the role to life itself. Just as the newborn infant does not enter the world as a person completely qualified for the role, neither is the emerging nurse fully qualified for the selected role. Both the newborn and the new nurse have major tasks to complete in order to function effectively. The creativity used to become effective is an essential element in achieving the goals that the newborn and the new nurse face. In addition, the process of creating the person or nurse is ongoing and is influenced by the environment that enriches or impinges on the developing person. The newborn, born with physical defects, needs to expend additional energy during the process of creation in order to compensate for the physical disability. The nurse, faced with creating a broader person in a helping role, expends more energy to become a self worthy of the chosen role. One can hypothesize that the greater the odds placed against the newborn or emerging nurse the greater is the need to use creativity during the process of creation of the personal self. The person who is able to use creativity effectively is in an advantaged position and will probably create a personal self that is capable of achieving high levels of excellence. This hypothesis does not include an assumption that anyone becomes competent without hard work and persistence, however. Even the most advantaged person undergoes periods of frustration and self-doubt during the creation process.

A tenet is postulated that the man or woman that enters the nursing profession, having a strong sense of personal self, will have less difficulty transcending the hurdles that need to be overcome to become a nurse in the purest sense of the word—nurturer. The strong personal self is then nurtured in the ways of the profession and results in a unification of the personal and professional self.

The inclusion of creativity into the creation of individuals provides for a wide range of individual persons capable of achieving the same professional goals. It is good to have distinct, humane people assume the responsibility for a profession. The distinctly different people all make important contributions to the nursing profession. The act of becoming a self-actualized nurse is not built upon conformity but upon a keenly aware and sensitive self as person. Being self-actualized is being well integrated.

Being integrated helps the nurse to function effectively in the chosen role. However, being integrated does not guarantee that nurses will act ethically and morally in all situations. Nurturance of integrated persons, therefore, requires that the person be exposed to ethical and moral principles that can be assimilated into the personality structure of individuals and expressed as morally and ethically sound nursing practice.

The following exercises relate to raising the level of consciousness about the way the nurse as person influences nursing practice.

EXERCISES

EXERCISE 1:

Write all the attributes you possess as a person. Have another person write all the attributes that they perceive you possess as a person. Compare the lists and discuss any discrepancies in the two lists.

EXERCISE 2:

Write a paragraph about the uniqueness you possess as a person. Then explore ways you can use this uniqueness in your nursing practice.

EXERCISE 3:

Design a profile of an "ideal self." Now star elements in the profile that you presently possess. Ask yourself if there are additional elements in the profile that you wish to cultivate. Encircle these elements. Make a plan for achieving your goal to develop these elements.

EXERCISE 4:

Examine a recent interaction with an individual or group. Were there positive elements of your personal self in the interaction? Were there negative elements of personal self in the interaction? Were all of your personal responses appropriate for professional interactions? If not, which ones need to be changed?

EXERCISE 5:

Recall a recent happy experience. What elements made it happy? Can these same elements be integrated into professional nursing practice to improve the quality of nursing practice?

DISCUSSION

These exercises attempt to stress the importance of the personal self to the profession of nursing. The activities can be used to strengthen the connections between personal and professional roles.

Behavioral Guidelines

Early writings related to ethics in nursing clearly identified acceptable and nonacceptable behaviors for a nurse. Today, there are limited explicit guidelines for behavior, and emerging nurses are vulnerable because of the lack of concensus among nurses regarding behaviors that are expected and rewarded. The seeming lack of established behaviors associated with practice results in a wide variability of exhibited behaviors being demonstrated and tolerated and apparently being acceptable. This situation can result in confusion as emerging nurses have to try to decide which behaviors are encouraged or condoned by the group that she/he is presently in association with. The situation is compounded by the fact that modern culture does not have any clearly identified shared ethical attitudes and values that help to provide direction for behavior. Therefore, the emerging nurse is left to create his/her own set of values regarding nursing without the aide of an adequate knowledge base or substantial experience. The difficult choices in relation to behavior that the emerging nurse needs to make relate to:

1) whether to be caring in practice,
2) whether to be authoritarian in practice,
3) whether to smile freely at clients,
4) whether to maintain adequate distance from clients,
5) whether to express personal feelings,

6) whether to follow the peers' behavior in the situation no matter what that behavior is,

7) whether to use creativity in practice or to follow the status quo,

8) whether to lead or to follow,

9) whether to support the ideals of the professional organization,

10) whether to be loyal to the organization or to the profession if there are conflicts between the two,

11) whether to withdraw from or participate in conflicts that arise,

12) whether to continue to study the literature after graduation or to learn only by experience,

13) whether to discard idealism in favor of realism,

14) whether to support activities that advance the profession, such as nursing research, or choose to ignore them.

When there are hazy standards of behavior, the nurse has no operational code of behavior to follow and lacks direction for adequate decision-making. When a person is confronted with this experience, he/she calls on the unconscious to resolve the conflict. The unconscious control approximates the life experiences the nurse encountered during his/her developmental stages. It is easy to hypothesize that, when facing crisis situations, nurses might resign from their positions, become angry, withdraw, confront the situation, cope with it successfully, and so forth. The wide range of behaviors exhibited in the culture at large are likely to be exhibited in the culture of nursing. In an earlier period, the nurses' behavior was influenced by the dictated behaviors of the profession. Today, the nurse is allowed to avoid resolving conflicts by changing positions or changing behavior. This behavior is an example of the nurse responding to the crisis of the moment rather than looking at self and feelings to explain the emotional stress that is related to the immediate crisis.

Gaining Insight

As nursing evolves into a dynamic and powerful force within the health care system, it is imperative that nurses develop insights into self and incorporate these personal insights within the profession. A sense of purpose and idealism needs to be re-established so that evolving nurses know the behaviors that are associated with the profession and are able to use these behaviors to help clients maintain or restore equilibrium and to promote the nursing profession as a caring humanistic enterprise.

Positive and possibility thinking in the mass literature is connected with success. There are many popular books that transmit this message. Browsing through the bookshelves of stores, bold letters jump out and promise instant success. Unfortunately, the success gained through these volumes is often limited to the author who merrily carries the profits to the bank, unaware of the outcomes of his/her prophesy to the consumer. The failure of the book in guaranteeing instant success relates to the unlikeliness of any one factor to possess the ability to achieve a goal as spectacular as the printed word boldly suggests: THINK POSITIVE, BE SUCCESSFUL; POSSIBILITY THINKING, SUCCESS IN THE ORGANIZATION. Success is intimately associated with the person's personality. Personality is extremely complex. A book can serve as a catalyst to instant success in some persons who willingly part with their money, but it probably will be a financial bomb for many persons who remove it from the shelf. The psychology of advertising proves to be more successful than the writer's message in many person's life scripts. Despite the failure rate, people continue to try to buy easy solutions to life's trials and tribulations. Purchasing another disappointment seems to be easier than constructively dealing with personal limitations and feelings that might lead to insights about self that influence personal and professional success or failure. The books often provide the reader with knowledge without insight, only half of the prescription needed for self-improvement, self-motivation, and self-fulfillment. There is apparently no end to the hope that major decisions and accomplishments can be achieved by purchasing a simple dehydrated form that needs only to be watered to spring forth as a million dollar adventure. Nothing can be farther from the truth. Success takes hard work and a combination of many factors in order to become reality. While books can be a vital element in the process of nurturing persons as persons, they cannot be delegated the total responsibility for the important growing, maturing, and rewarding experience. The individual person must assume the major responsibility for experiencing the self as self.

Gaining insight involves becoming aware of something within ourselves that we previously submerged in our unconscious mind. Gaining insight involves getting to know others and nature in a new and interesting way. Gaining insight requires an honest reappraisal of the way we perceive life and living. Gaining insight necessitates a change in perspective, a restructuring of the way that life's events and happenings are viewed. Gaining insight requires a reassessment of the values placed on people, places, and things. Gaining insight requires the discarding of outdated information in exchange for new and innovative possibilities. Gaining insight accentuates the need to be a vital and dynamic force in the systems of which we are a part: family, church, clubs, organizations, professions, and so forth. Yes, gaining insight requires a restructuring of reality, affectively and cognitively, and involves areas that impact the total personality.

Creativity and People

There are a number of experts who have contributed to the understanding of the process of creativity and its relevance to the becoming of individuals. Some of the ideas of these authorities are included to show the relationship of creativity to the enhancing of the nurse as a person.

The creative person, according to MacKinnon,[1] is one who reconciles the opposites of expert knowledge and childlike naive wonder and freshness of perceptions in their desire to look at problems in new ways. He suggests that creative persons are more likely to be open to their own feelings and emotions. In addition, creative persons have wide-ranging interests and possess a sensitive intellect.

The self is actualized through experiencing in a variety of ways during the process of living. As a person, to view living as a creative process requires viewing love, work, and life as an art.[2] To bring greater meaning into life it is necessary to live each day anticipating a fuller, more expression-filled existence. The creative individual is continually undergoing an unfolding process. The unfolding process is essential to the growth of individuals in their movement towards their goal of self-actualization. Maslow's[3] hierachy of needs is useful in understanding this concept. A person who is striving to achieve basic needs is in a disadvantaged position to express creativity. Too much energy is being expended on achieving needs essential for survival. A person who has achieved basic needs is better able to move towards self-actualization.

Moustakas[4] suggests that to be creative one needs to experience life in his/her unique way, perceiving from within while drawing upon one's own resources and capabilities to respond with a whole array of emotions ranging from joy through sorrow. Searching into one's self allows creative potential to emerge. It is the deep emergence into self that results in one truly getting to know oneself. Or stated another way, it is the revealing of one's self to oneself. This process helps the person to be honest and consistent with his/her own feelings and devoted to living a full and effective life. Moustakas believes that being able to respond to inner and outer resources is essential if one is to be capable of creative expression. Creativity involves either a deep involvement of one person with another or the involvement of a person with raw materials of nature and life.

May[5] suggests that it is necessary for people to rid themselves of inhibitions in order to free themselves to be truly creative. He suggests that people need to enjoy the tension associated with new situations in order to be able to approach them creatively.

The world we live in is fashioned by reason, imagination and emotions. An assumption is made that the world would be a better place to live in if human beings think and feel deeply and intentionally influence the form the world will take. The potential to influence the world is held by each of us. The interrelationships we have with our world are meaningful, and these interrelationships bring meaning to life. Creativity is part of experiencing and is present in the drama which encompasses self-world relationships.

> *Every man is the creature of the age in which he lives; very few are able to raise themselves above the ideas of the times.*
>
> Voltaire

> *Had I been present at the creation of the world I would have proposed some improvements.*
>
> Alfonso X

Moustakas[6] cautions that during the process of creating it is not possible to be concerned about other persons' reactions to the creation. If the creator takes time to focus on other people's reactions, it interferes with the process of creation. In other words, the process of creation necessitates the creator's undivided attention.

Maslow[3] highlights an interesting proposition when he suggests that sensory deprivation, to a healthy person, is both pleasing and frightening. He bases this on the idea that when the outer world is cut off, the inner world comes to consciousness. A close proximity to the inner world is more acceptable to healthy persons than to unhealthy persons. Therefore, healthy people are able to benefit from and enjoy periods of sensory deprivation that are poorly tolerated by unhealthy people. These periods of intermittent sensory deprivation can be utilized to think creatively, to nurture self-fulfillment, and to recharge the fatigued self.

The person in touch with himself/herself feels comfortable to express his identity, to be free, to be self. The self-assurance which accompanies this state of being provides adequate protection from persons who express doubt about experiencing life in this way. The creative person meets many disbelievers who tend to question and disvalue the sense of being oneself, of knowing where one is headed, and being free to question without fear of seeming unknowledgeable or unsure. People who are less secure about themselves tend to want everyone else to know that they harbor doubts about the creative person's ideas, and they take every opportunity to make these reservations known. The person in touch with himself/herself takes this situation in stride and continues to function effectively, undaunted by other people's desires to stifle creative impulses and transform them into more logical, traditional forms. Moustakas notes that a person cannot totally destroy his/her real self in order to please others. In a world where so much energy is focused on directing how persons will behave, it is difficult to keep one's own identity free from the influence of directing that is based on conformity.

The psychology of the creative is really feminine psychology,
a fact which proves that creative work grows out of the
unconscious depths, indeed out of the region of the mothers.

Carl Jung

Martindale[7] notes that creative persons do not tolerate simple distractions readily. However, they possess a preference for complicated distractions as well as complicated attractions. This is illustrated by the creative person's preference for complex designs, asymmetry, ambiguous and odd designs as opposed to the simple, familiar designs often preferred by less creative persons. These identified preferences seem consistent with the spontaneous, uncontrolled nature of inspiration which is associated with the generation of new and nontraditional ideas.

Martindale[7] noted that creative persons describe themselves by using the adjectives *enthusiastic, assertive,* and *impulsive* while noncreative persons choose the adjectives *contented, conventional, virtuous,* and *rational* to describe themselves. The adjectives selected by created persons clearly document the need for nonconventional environments to facilitate creative behavior. Many traditional environments tend to squelch enthusiasm and impulsive and assertive behavior.

The freedom to be one's self emerges as being paramount to being creative. The creative person tends to be relatively at ease with self. This at-ease posture allows a person to trust and to love. Basic to trust and love of others is trust and love of self. Successful achievement of self-trust and love allows the person to gain self-confidence. Self-trust and love provide a sense of security that is needed to handle the feeling states that evolve from a diversity of human experiences and interactions.

Human Interactions

Human interactions are common every day occurrences. As such, they need to be continually strengthened so they provide greater satisfaction for the persons involved in them. Few persons would deny that communication is more complicated in a technological society. At the same time that advances are made in all areas of communication techniques, there is a decrease in the ability for individuals to communicate effectively with one another, as documented by the increase in divorce rate in this country, by the high incidence of persons seeking professional counseling, and by the self-awareness conferences focusing on improving personal communication.

Unfortunately, there are no simple solutions or complicated machinery to improve the quality of human interactions. Only hard work and persistence on the part of each of us will result in this outcome. There must be a desire on the part of each participant to improve the quality of human interactions to have it happen.

It is common to hear phrases like "being together," "I need to get my head on straight," "getting it all together," "getting my act together," "getting in touch with myself," "finding out who I am," "finding where I'm coming from," "getting in touch with my feelings," "doing my own thing." These phrases are associated with the self-awareness movement that is infiltrating or sweeping society. There seems to be greater need expressed by persons to fully understand themselves. People are eager to feel they are important as people as well as in their diversified roles of mother, father, engineer, nurse, commuter, student, and so forth. People seem anxious to benefit from life experiences and to make meaning out of them. There is an openness to explore new life experiences and an increased effort to make these experiences meaningful and growth-producing. The self-awareness movement is not without its critics, however. Some persons feel that the increased emphasis on self is resulting in a decreased awareness of the needs of a broader society. In this discussion, the emphasis on self is supported on the basis that increased self-awareness and fulfillment will benefit society at large, not weaken it.

The following quotation by Merton[8] expresses the intent of this discussion.

> He who attempts to act and do things for others or for the world without deepening his own self-understanding, freedom, integrity, and capacity to love will not have anything to give others. He will communicate to them nothing but the contagion of his own obsessions, his aggressiveness, his ego-centered ambitions, his delusions about ends and means, his doctrinaire prejudices and ideas.

The person sincerely desiring to increase the worth of self is encouraged to have a diversified group of friends and acquaintances to interact with. Persons representing various disciplines, interesting people in the arts as well as the sciences, will bring new insights and awakenings to the person. An attempt is made to keep the mind responding to a broad range of topics. In this day of specialization, it is too easy to narrow down the mind's output by focusing on only a narrow range of ideas and experiences. To use a somewhat over-used cliche, a specialist is someone who knows more and more about less and less. A broader prepared group of acquaintances makes it difficult to respond to only one area of interest.

This suggestion does not propose that other nurses are not broadly educated people with a wide range of interests. It does, however, take into account that when a group is composed solely with nurses there is an increased possibility that professional activities will be discussed. Including people from other disciplines in the group tends to keep us honest with ourselves. In a group situation these people will not tolerate nurses keeping their interesting personal selves submerged below their professional selves.

Awareness

In his book, Stevens[9] identifies three zones of awareness. These include awareness of the outside world, awareness of the inside world, and awareness of fantasy activity. Awareness of the outside and inside worlds relate to happenings in the present. Awareness of the outside world includes sensory contact with objects and events. Awareness of the inside world includes sensory contacts with inner events.

Heintz, Fieweger, and Fitzgerald[10] suggest that the qualities of awareness include 1) openness, 2) awareness of detail, and 3) empathy. The openness allows the person to take from the surroundings a variety of experiences which are interpreted in accordance with individual perceptions. The way a person perceives the environment is closely connected to his/her ability to feel the situation or empathize with it. The awareness ability is facilitated by being conscious of detail and paying increased attention to life experiences. May[5] suggests that for a person to live with sensitivity in this period, when everything seems to be in limbo, requires courage. Sensitivity is an essential component of awareness.

Flach[11] identifies a four-step creative process that can be used to increase personal awareness: 1) preparation, 2) incubation, 3) illumination, and 4) verification. In the preparation stage, the person becomes fully engrossed with the subject. In the second stage, the subject is allowed to pass from the conscious mind to the preconscious mind. In the third stage the conscious mind is filled with new possibilities for resolving dilemmas, and in the fourth stage the new possibilities are tested in reality. The four-step process is similiar in methodology to the five step creative problem-solving process identified in Chapter 5. However, the terminology suggested by Flach seems to be closely associated with the personal emphasis in this chapter. It is easy to envision the person as preparing for personal change, thinking (or incubating) about it, gaining insights (illumination), and then trying out the possibilities (verification).

The four-step process is hypothesized as more *person-directed* than *thing* or *place-directed.* The five-step process is more thing or place-directed than person-directed.*

Therefore, in this chapter, the four-step process of Flach is proposed as a viable alternative to the five-step process. The following scenario serves as an example:

Mary is 20 years old. She is a sophomore at a large university that offers a four year baccalaureate degree in nursing. She is studying conscientiously but receives low C's in course work instead of the A's she consistently received in her small high school. The recurring question she asks herself is whether or not to quit nursing. Mary alternatedly answers the question with a yes or a no. Despite her simple answers she does not feel comfortable to act upon her choice. She clearly indicates, to herself, an ambiguity about the situation. She needs to redefine the question and try to find a more creative alternative.

Preparation. Mary goes beyond the one-track questions and answer modality and completely submerges herself in the problem which she redefines as: What do I want to do with my life? The broader problem statement propelled Mary into a consideration of the following.

a) do I prefer work with people or things?
b) do I want a nursing career enough to risk temporary failures?
c) do I know myself well enought to understand other people?
d) would I be happier at a smaller university or college?
e) should I take some time off and explore the world before selecting a career?
f) do I have a handle on what it means to be a woman?
g) have I nurtured or inhibited relationships with peers?
h) am I a dependent or independent person?
i) do I prefer to be alone or with others?
j) have I thoroughly explored choices open to me?
k) am I deliberately getting lower grades so I can fail?
l) what role models do I identify with?

Mary spent many hours trying to sort out the questions and answers that emerged from her exploration of the redefined question. After she made a thorough analysis she returned to her studies and tried to separate herself from the problem temporarily (incubation stage).

A week went by and on a Tuesday night Mary was awakened from a sound sleep by a dream. In her dream, she was sitting silently next to the bed of an elderly woman who was dying. She was holding the woman's hand and sharing in the moment of death, a moment prized by the woman and Mary.

Mary sat up startled and brought the dream to consciousness. She suddenly realized that she had the answer to her question. She must stay in nursing and persevere until she achieved her goal. The intense submersion in her problem finally produced a more realistic answer to her question (illumination stage). Now Mary faced the reality of trying out the solution. She must achieve satisfactory grades in order to fulfill her career goals. The renewed commitment to her goals would help to make her desires possible, but only time will provide evidence of her success or failure (verification stage).

This approach allowed Mary to leave the logical domain of thinking and use the preconscious (creative thinking) to get in touch with her feelings about herself as a person and about nursing and life. She was freed from producing an immediate response to her dilemma and provided with an opportunity to use introspection, disciplined thinking, and time to help to provide direction for her future course of action. She was not afraid to examine problems that required her to explore areas within herself that produced discomfort, pain, satisfaction, or concern. She willingly submerged herself in the personal problem to arrive at a decision that escaped her in the past.

The following exercises will enhance awareness of the environment.

EXERCISES

EXERCISE 1:

Explore the environment. Select something that symbolizes why you chose the dress or suit you are wearing today. Then explain the symbolism to another.

EXERCISE 2:

Explore your environment and select something that symbolizes why you chose nursing as a profession. Then explain the symbolism to another. Note: If you do not have another person to share the experience with, sit in front of a mirror and explain it to your image.

EXERCISE 3:

Snap photographs of scenes that have meaning to you. When the pictures are ready, ask what it is in the picture that made you take this particular image. Note: If you do not have a camera or do not want to wait to develop the picture, you can form an imaginary camera with your hands and snap an imaginary picture in the same way. Explain what is in the picture and the meaning it has for you.

DISCUSSION

In the three exercises the participant is using symbolism as a stimulus to creativity and creative expression. It is helpful to provide "crutches" for people to use to help them exercise inner thoughts and ideas; these exercises are suggested crutches.

Awareness must be developed. There must be a deliberate attempt to discard habits and attitudes that interfere with the process. One attitude that inhibits the ability to be aware is the feeling that other people will think we are silly, immature, or different. It takes a great deal of courage to allow oneself the freedom to explore with openness when there are so many critics ready to criticize and pass judgment. It also takes courage to try new things rather than responding to situations in the traditional way. It is well to adopt an attitude that it is possible to do and see things differently and that there is merit in doing so. Assume a posture that it is possible to find out more than is presently known and it is possible to learn more about self when exploring without controls.

Another opportunity to increase awareness of the environment is by witnessing happenings; while the brain registers the observations, describe verbally what is being witnessed. Describing situations verbally helps to improve one's powers of observations because hearing the description increases awareness of details that are included or omitted from the description of the observations.

While increasing awareness, the observer needs to be thinking about the future as well as the past and present. Material gathered from observations needs to be evaluated in terms of its future use. The more ways that information can be manipulated for potential use, the better. Therefore, at the same time one focuses on being a better person, he/she is also searching for ways to be a better professional, neighbor, citizen, and so forth.

There are some simple exercises which help to foster general awareness. Try some of the following.

EXERCISES

EXERCISE 1:

Take a large sheet of plain paper and create with finger paints. Deliberately cue in on how it feels to your fingers, your palms, the whole hand. Look at the design and think if it has special meaning, focus on the colors and what meanings they have, what flowed through your mind while you were involved in the activity, did your thoughts change at all, is there any "message" from the experience?

EXERCISE 2:

Take a piece of silly putty. Close your eyes. Keep changing its form. As you do this deliberately focus on the changing object. Focus on how it feels and smells. Fantasize new ways that it could be used.

EXERCISE 3:

Take clay. Close your eyes and manipulate it. Then open your eyes and manipulate it. Focus on shape, depth, width, texture. Periodically ask what it exemplifies. How does it feel? Does it feel like anything else you felt recently? What is it most like? Why did you choose that particular object? What is it most unlike? Why did you choose that particular object? Can you make any connections between the clay and the object it is most like or unlike? Did you like the feeling aroused when manipulating the clay? Does it feel "emotionally" any different than it feels to your hands? If you like the feeling, how can you keep it? If you dislike the feeling, how can you get rid of it?

EXERCISE 4:

Select an animal you would like to be. Act out being that animal. Explore why you chose the animal, how it felt to be the animal, and what messages you received from the experience.

EXERCISE 5:

Select something from nature (ie, lightning, moon, stars, etc). Act out being this part of nature. Think why you liked this role, why you disliked the role, why you chose it. Did you learn anything about yourself by the exercise? Are there other things you need to explore in relation to ideas that developed from the exercise?

EXERCISE 6:

Use the tips of your fingers and deliberately explore different skin surfaces of your body while your eyes are closed. Pay special attention to rough spots, soft spots, hairy spots, moles, fingernails, etc. Pay attention to the feelings that emerge as you focus on particular areas. Are there areas that you enjoyed touching more than others? Are there areas you avoided touching? Are there areas you disliked touching? Ask yourself why? Try to force yourself to discover new reasons for your willingness or hesitance to explore your body. Then close your eyes and explore again. Next compare the two explorations. Did you learn anything new about yourself by doing this exercise?

EXERCISE 7:

Take a piece of fruit such as an apple, lemon, or orange from a bag of fruit. Get completely in touch with the fruit. Use all your senses with the exception of taste. Put your fruit back in the bag and shake it up. Then without the use of sight, reach in the bag and take your piece of fruit out. Did you get your fruit? How did you know to select it? If you missed, try the exercise again. Train your senses to work to identify details. If you are successful, reward yourself through your taste sense.

DISCUSSION

Exercises 1 through 7 utilize the senses to trigger inner thoughts and ideas. The exercises are vehicles for making connections between ideas. At the same time, the exercises try to get the participant to understand self and pay attention to things that are liked and things that are disliked. There is a deliberate attempt to get the participant fully involved in the exploration process and to bring unconscious thoughts to the conscious mind.

These exercises can be done singly or as a group. They can be repeated on more than one occasion with only slight variations in the questions that are asked.

Personal Goals

Persons need both short term and long term goals; however, the long term goals are the dominant ones. Short term goals that are not consistent with a person's long term goals need to be aborted to avoid dissatisfaction later. Short term goals bring immediate gratification. However, if they run counter to important long term goals, short term goals are not worth the emotional investment they necessitate. Even a large number of short term accomplishments does not yield the same personal satisfaction as achieving a significant long term goal. Therefore, all short term goals must be congruent with specified long term goals to provide continual gratification and satisfaction. A good way to examine the congruence between short and long term goals is to write them out and compare them. Writing out goals is a better strategy than just thinking about goals, as a better analysis can be achieved. The goals can be assessed and thoughtful reflection can take place.

The goals set by an individual are unique to that individual. Goals are based on a person's own needs and values and reflect the choices which best represent his/her personal desires. Goals which are not fully selected or which are based on the other person's values can result in decisions which are not the best alternative(s) for the individual. Therefore, it is important to continually assess if the selected goals truly reflect the values which will result in the greatest personal satisfaction to the individual.

In order to truly be a fulfilled person it is necessary to ask searching questions related to the way choices are made and the way a particular action is chosen over other actions. In this process of self-questioning it is essential for the person to assess his/her degree of happiness. If a person is happy, why? If a person is not happy, then why not? Two exercises are provided to focus on the personal goals of individuals.

EXERCISES

EXERCISE 1:

Make three wishes that express desires you have for yourself. Write the three wishes on a piece of paper.

EXERCISE 2:

Think of a person that you would like to trade places with. Write down all the facts you can about the person you selected.

DISCUSSION

After the participant writes out the material, he/she is asked to think why the particular wish or person was chosen and to decide how this information could be used to derive self-happiness. He/she is also advised to think about the degree of discrepancy between the person he/she is now and the person that he/she would be if those ideas were incorporated.

Creative Experiences

The aesthetic mode of human experience is not only nice but necessary. Broudy[12] clarifies the difference between the aesthetic mode of experience and artistic activity by explaining that the aesthetic mode of experience is the generic activity that everyone participates in, while artistic activity is a species of aesthetic experience reserved for a select group.

> *He is the greatest artist who has embodied, in the sum of his*
> *works, the greatest number of the greatest ideas.*
>
> John Ruskin

People vary greatly in the amount of self-renewal they derive from attending creative experiences. A visit to the art museum opens vistas for some persons while others do not see any merit in viewing art. Various forms of dance are selected by some persons to help to awaken their inner feelings while others find dance as a complete waste of time and do not respond to the message it provides. Music provides hours of relaxation and results in creative expression for those who appreciate its value while others do not respond to the messages it transmits. Each art form known to man can stimulate some persons while leaving other persons untouched. Exposure to any of these mediums has the potential to arouse a variety of responses: exhilaration, excitement, motivation, stimulation, intrigue, or relaxation. In addition, the emotions of frustration, anger, disappointment, uneasiness, and dissatisfaction can also be aroused by some creative offerings. If the arts and humanities have the possibility of arousing such a wide variation of emotions, why are they chosen by so many people to fill their recreational hours? The answer is quite simple. The arts and humanities provide individuals with opportunities to fantasize, imagine, pretend, relive, anticipate, and create life experiences that provide an escape from the day to day existence that they lead.

Creative experiences provide an opportunity for people to come closer to the world that the artist sees as reality. These creative experiences make it possible for the observer to be involved with the feelings expressed via the art form by persons who possess proven creative ability. This exposure to creative experiences often stimulates creative productivity in the observer by triggering inner thoughts. The magic-like quality involved in this process is not fully understood. The emergence of creative productivity is possibly associated with the potential for creative experiences to induce connections between the conscious and unconscious mind and vice versa. The ability for some persons to benefit from these experiences while others do not is too complex to discuss in its entirety. However, May[5] provides one explanation that seems quite logical. He suggests that when viewing an art form, the viewer experiences a new moment of sensibility. The experience results in new visions which arise from associations stored in the subconscious mind. The new vision of the observer is awakened by observing the creation of the artist. In this instance, the response to a creative experience of another person helps to rouse a creative act from the viewer. An important point to remember is that mere exposure to a creative product of another does not always result in the release of creative potential in the observer. However, there is a possibility for this to happen, but there is no predictable cause and effect reaction produced.

> *Art flourishes where there is a sense of adventure, a sense of nothing having been done before, of complete freedom to experiment; but when caution comes in you get repetition, and repetition is the death of art.*
>
> Alfred Whitehead

The creative experiences one chooses to attend can become habit forming. When an experience becomes a habit, it is less likely to result in stimulating creative potential. Attending a variety of creative experiences is more likely to stimulate creative behavior than attending repeated sessions of the same creative experience. However, some persons attend the same medium and work at perfecting their understanding of it. This type of intense involvement with the medium is sometimes capable of motivating the person to search for the best expression of his/her own creative potential. The creative expression which arises from this situation is probably explained on the basis of the active role of the participant in the creative experience which is more beneficial than a passive role for encouraging the observer to produce.

The degree of creativity possessed by the participant is also an important variable when persons are confronted with creative experiences. The person that is highly creative seems to derive more stimulation from creative experiences than persons who are less creative in their manner. The wide variation in response, based on creative ability, makes it difficult to draw generalizations about the advantages to be accrued by individuals from involvement with creative experiences.

Many creative experiences succeed in putting meaning into our lives.

Attendance at selected creative experiences can bring joy, fulfillment, and a deepening sense of being. May[5] refers to creative experiences as original creativity of the spirit, an appropriate title for sure.

Attendance at something is not a requirement for having a creative experience. Many books provide magnificent creative experiences. Writers share a variety of ideas that can activate creative expression in the reader. The value of reading can be increased by reading out loud. Somehow the audible expression of the written message increases the creative stimulation that reading produces. Poems are an excellent source of inspiration. The poems that encourage self-awareness can be read in minimal time, some in less than five minutes. These messages can have a dramatic impact on the individual. Personal preference will determine what written material is most inspirational. Developing the habit of reading extensively is congruent with creative expression. The ideas of others help to trigger stored associations in the brain. These associations can result in unique creative responses.

> *The writer is the engineer of the human soul.*
>
> Joseph Stalin

> *In some ways, certain books are more powerful by far than any battle.*
>
> Henry Wallace

To name all the things in life that have the ingredients for raising creative potential in each individual would be impossible. Some persons respond to pets, some to children, some to riding on a bus, some to the sound of a train, and so forth. Each person needs to identify the creativity stimulators in his/her own environment and use the stimulators effectively.

The values derived from creative experiences go beyond the rewards gained by the personal self. A person's personal and professional life are closely interwoven. A person that feels good about self is more likely to be successful in a professional role. Therefore it is essential to focus attention on the personal self and to delineate ways that creativity relates to that personal self in order to understand the ways that creativity pertains to the professional roles that the nurse assumes.

Maslow[13] suggests that the concept of the self-actualizing person and the concept of creativeness are probably synonomous. His hypothesis is intriguing as it tends to elevate the importance of creativity to the nursing profession. The lives of people who are able to achieve a high level of integration of self are likely to also be people who exhibit creativity. The self-actualized person tends to be creative in all the roles he/she assumes. Therefore, a self-actualized person is likely to be a creative nurse as well as a creative person. The improvement of the person, in general, helps to improve the specific or specialized areas of functioning of the person, as well. It appears that the more creative a person becomes the more likely the person will gain in every sphere of life.

Self-actualization in relation to nursing is the act of setting out to be a first rate nurse and working intensely to achieve this goal. Self-actualization is the act of becoming a first-rate nurse and not being satisfied with becoming anything less than the best nurse that it is possible to become.

Creative Games

DiCyan[14] stresses the importance of creative games to generate creativity to find solutions to problems. He notes that competition is not the goal of these games but rather the games are left unstructured to allow the creative potential of the players to emerge. The games, free of directions, offer opportunities for the participants to infer the steps necessary to reach a successful conclusion. Directionless activity frees the mind to go off in new and unusual directions. Children freely express their creativity through games. Adults, however, are restrained and frequently cannot use the same vehicle to stimulate creativity as reflected in the following example.

> On one of the evaluations of a creative problem solving workshop,[15] the following suggestion was made, "Cut out all the games and really teach how to be creative. Without the games, there was only three hours of content on creative problem solving."

Despite our attempts to help this participant conceptualize the entire process involved in stimulating creative behavior, he did not see the relevance of participating in creative games.

> *All ordinary expression may be explained causally, but creative expression which is the absolute contrary of ordinary expression, will be forever hidden from human knowledge.*
>
> Carl Jung

Products of Creativity

MacKinnon[1] makes a distinction between two types of creative products: scientific and artistic. He suggests that artistic creative products are ones that originate from the inner feelings and emotions of the creator, while scientific creative products are not related to the person's inner being. In the latter, the creative person serves as a liaison between external needs and goals. The artistic creative product is a reflection of the creator as a person while the scientific creative product is relatively free from the personal being of the creator. MacKinnon adds, however, that the affective aspects of creation are probably expressed in some forms of scientific creative products just as in artistic creative products. The creative products with the least personal inner involvement of the creator are advanced technology and inventions.

The creative person enjoys turning out creative products. These products are original, useful, and sometimes novel. The quality of usefulness is essential if a product is to meet the criteria of a creative product. Artistic products traditionally associated with creativity are paintings, music, dance, and architecture. However, products of creativity are not limited to these traditional artistic productions. Limiting creative products to these high achievements is to ignore the value of less dramatic but significant creative outputs.

An objective of the creator is to identify problems. The creator breaks the problems down into smaller more manageable problems and generates ideas for solving the problem. A creative product is the outcome. Criteria for evaluating creative products are as follows: they are original; they possess aesthetic qualities; and they evolve from a thorough exploration of the mind involving ideation, imagination, and interaction of the conscious and the unconscious mind.

MacKinnon[1] suggests that creative products are not limited to the arts and sciences, and that some people are creative products themselves. He attributes the potential for persons to be creative products to climates that allow persons to develop and express their personal lives in a creative way. The creative person "as product" is helpful in solving the problems of business, education, political, and military establishments. The person, as creative product, plays an extremely valuable role in perceiving needed change and in exploring alternatives available to make the changes. In order for the person to act in this capacity, the environment must tolerate flexibility and change and value the contributions made by the "creative product."

The act of creation is an intense experience. It does not happen easily. The person who is involved in a creative act must be deeply immersed in the process. As May[5] notes, it is an intensive encounter that eventually results in a creative act. This encounter fully absorbs the person. There is a heightened awareness on the part of the individual from the intense commitment to the creative act. This total immersion in the task eventually produces the joy that accompanies the experience of self-actualization. Creation requires a blend between intensive work and moments of relaxation. Unfortunately, there is no magic formula for determining the proportions of each that are needed to result in a successful experience of creating.

Creativity does not take place in a vacuum; it is part and parcel of things the creator already suspects or knows. There is variability in the way ideas emerge. Ideas may flow freely early in the morning after a refreshing night's sleep. Sometimes the person is awakened from a sound sleep by ideas. The ideas must be captured and expressed to take full advantage of the results of the conscious and unconscious levels of awareness coming together. When ideas emerge they need to be written down immediately. The conscious mind cannot be trusted to remember the ideas after they emerge. Descriptions have been given to express the vividness with which break-throughs in thinking appear; it is likened to a new life, or being bright, clear and having freshness.

One prescription for making the best use of the unconscious mind is to provide for periods of solitude. The act of being alone, free from noise and distractions, is important to some persons for bringing messages from the unconscious. The periods of solitude allow the ideas and insights stored in the unconscious mind to emerge. In a more hectic, noisy setting, the unconscious mind is unable to be utilized effectively, and ideas are lost or remain stored in the unconscious mind until the environment is more conducive to idea generation.

> *A man can be himself only so long as he is alone; and, if he does not love solitude, he will not love freedom; for it is only when he is alone that he is really free.*
>
> Arthur Schopenhauer

Once a breakthrough comes, it seems so logical, so true. At the moment that the idea emerges, it seems to be the most appropriate solution to the problem. The breakthrough raises the question in the creator's mind of why such an obvious solution was not produced sooner. The reason the breakthrough took so long to come is probably associated with timing. Prior to this moment, substantial conscious level activity with the associated tension and constructive stress was inadequate to help the unconscious mind release the sought after ideas. An in-depth period of work was not completed prior to this time, therefore, the right answer did not emerge sooner. The quality of creative products is clearly associated with the ideation process which is associated with significant breakthroughs in traditional thinking.

The creative products needed in nursing, or for that matter any field, are frequently produced by thinkers from outside the field. A person with a new outlook is able to bring a repertoire of knowledge, combine it with imagination, and generate ideas which facilitate creative products useful in nursing practice. Many of the advances in the health field are creations of engineers or inventors who collaborate with health professionals to produce needed creative products. Examples of this are numerous: technology for monitoring acutely ill patients, controlling the amount of intravenous fluid, motorized wheelchairs, and so forth. An example of a creative product in the artistic domain in nursing is the Loeb Center for Nursing in New York. Lydia Hall, a nurse, envisioned a new milieu for delivery of nursing services and diligently worked to develop and implement her creative idea. The result is an artistic creative product. A center where nurses, in collaboration with clients, plan, implement, and supervise nursing care in a milieu conducive to the recovery from illness.

> *If a man will begin with certainties, he will end in doubts; but if he will be content to begin with doubts, he will end in certainties.*
>
> Francis Bacon

There are, undoubtedly, many creative products that are envisioned by nurses that are never produced. Ideas regarding creative products emerge at the most inopportune times. Therefore they are pushed out of conscious awareness. For example, while doing a procedure, a need is identified for a more adequate instrument or dressing but the time is not conducive for brainstorming the problem and generating alternatives acceptable for doing the procedure more effectively and efficiently. Instead of writing down the problem for later resolution, it is suppressed into the unconscious and forgotten. Ideas for creative products are too valuable to lose. They must be captured. Then, when the opportunity is more conducive the written problems are conveniently retrieved for creative attack by self or others. Being aware of and sensitive to problems is the first valuable step in producing a creative product. The nurse is in an advantaged position for identifying problems that are conducive to creative resolution and generation of valuable creative products which will simplify or facilitate nursing practice.

Programs for Expanding Self

There are numerous programs, offered yearly, that are available for expanding oneself as a person. These programs vary a great deal in content and format. Some of the personal expansion programs are integrated with other theory content offerings, while some programs are focused solely on personal development. The nurse has the opportunity to pursue brochures and identify programs that have the potential for nurturing creative behavior towards the improvement of self. The Creative Problem Solving Institute in Buffalo, New York, and its satellite programs in several states are examples of programs specifically geared for the purpose of enhancing creative potential of participants.

Other opportunities that may be appealing, based on individual preferences, include sensitivity programs; Eastern philosophies and practices such as meditation or yoga; consciousness raising programs; leadership facilitation seminars; self-awareness offerings; assertiveness training; extrasensory perception workshops; and programs related to psychic phenomena. This list is not meant to imply that it is necessary to attend a program to become creative; however, practicing creative thinking does result in generating more creative ability. Therefore, programs which deliberately focus on producing creative behavior are likely to stimulate additional interest and practice opportunities for those electing to attend them. Frequently, these programs result in the participant gaining new insights as opposed to absolute solutions to personal concerns. A word of caution is also necessary. Attendance at a conference is only valuable if energy is expended to continue the growth producing experiences in daily living. Re-entry into ordinary routines following these programs can be traumatic if a concerted effort is not made to bring consonance between the program and the world at large. This suggests that it is necessary to temper down the programs as they near completion and focus on every day life experiences in an attempt to make the experiences more meaningful. Conscious attention must be focused on experiences of the institute as well as life experiences if the full value of the workshop is to be realized.

Participants in programs value ongoing association with other creative people so reinforcement for creative behavior becomes an ongoing process. The ongoing association with other creative thinkers serves as an energizing force. There are peaks and valleys in creative productivity; association with other creative people tends to lessen the valleys and to increase the peaks.

Chapter 10

Nurturing Creative Faculty Facilitators

> *We must have teachers—a heroine in every classroom.*
>
> Fidel Castro

This section includes a discussion of the nurturing of creativity during the preparation of faculty facilitators as well as how to be a creative faculty facilitator. The following quote from an outstanding nurse educator highlights the essence of what this section attempts to convey.

> Nursing has for too long been guilty of promoting conformists and of being punitive to those who are innovative and creative. The field suffers from a dearth of persons whose motivations and discoveries have vitalized the profession....The demonstration of real leadership in nursing will come when those who are now leaders in the field identify, foster and promote the deliberate preparation of their successors.[1]

The work of Ackoff[2] in relation to preparing competent managers is relevant here. He identifies five C's essential to managers: competence, communicativeness, concern, courage, and creativity. Ackoff hypothesizes that teachers only attempt to teach students competence, communicativeness, and occasionally concern for others. These three essential properties only partially complete the list of properties he identifies as essential for being successful in management situations. The properties that he suggests teachers do not attempt to transmit to students are *courage* and *creativity.* He suggests that teachers omit these areas from the curriculum because many teachers believe these characteristics are innate and cannot be taught or learned. These areas, however, can be taught and learned, and students that are not exposed to them are deprived of an important part of their education. The criticism of teachers posed by Ackoff is a serious charge.

The role of the faculty facilitator is to discover the potential for creative expression in the learner and to nourish that potential to actualization. To do less will result in the profession losing some of the most valuable talent possessed by persons selecting the nursing profession. The way to nurture creative potential to fruition is to identify it early and to set an academic and social climate that is conducive to developing their potential. Faculty facilitators who wait for the creative potential to spring forth by itself run the risk of not developing the skills in students essential for becoming a truly creative person, a person capable of being a truly creative faculty facilitator after their graduation. The education of educators is an essential responsibility of the nursing profession. The standards set for educator's education influence the future quality of the profession. There are teaching strategies which facilitate the effective functioning of individual's selecting the dual roles of education and nursing. Exposure to these strategies are included within the educational preparation of future faculty facilitators to assure competence of the graduates of the program.

The faculty facilitator of future faculty facilitators encourages a questioning stance. Future faculty facilitators are encouraged to openly explore the ideas of the faculty facilitator and challenge and threaten the judgments he/she espouses. This continual probing of ideas to discover "new truths" is conducive to nurturing creativity. The *a-ha* experiences which evolve from this interaction with ideas are the true rewards generated from an educational process. During these interactions faculty facilitators and future faculty facilitators learn together. The gains derived from the experiences are extraordinary for both sets of actors. In this type of environment there tends to be an aura of mutual dissatisfaction with what presently is known that stimulates and motivates learning.

Creative students are not always a delight to have around. There will be periods when their eagerness to explore ideas is disruptive and uncomfortable for the faculty facilitator. However, standing back and giving them the freedom to do "their own thing" will often result in original solutions to problems. Preparation of future faculty facilitators, patterned on questioning and idea generation, is a logical alternative to the traditional teacher-directed methods currently in use in many educator preparation programs in nursing.

One goal of the educational process is to keep learners a little frustrated so they try to overcome the frustration by using their abilities to solve problems. The uneasiness produced by frustration results in maximizing their potential for producing creative solutions to the problems they face. The principle of inducing frustration is especially relevant when dealing with intellectually gifted students. The education of educators is often focused on educating the gifted members of the profession, so this principle is very essential when planning curriculums for this group.

> *Consistency is the quality of a stagnant mind.*
>
> John Sloan

The perpetuation of a profession is a big responsibility, and persons assuming this responsibility should be persons with exceptional ability and personal qualifications. The faculty facilitator is accountable for preparing students to practice safely, effectively, caringly, and competently in the professions of nursing and education. The role of a nursing educator cannot be assumed without including competence in education as well as nursing. Because nursing personnel frequently function in life-death situations, it is crucial that the preparation of all levels of students be accomplished in a responsible way. Faculty facilitator preparation is intimately connected with this responsibility. An educational program which prepares the potential faculty facilitator with a scientific knowledge base is strengthened by the inclusion of strategies to advance the art of nursing. The emphasis of the educational program must be on preparing faculty facilitators to meet the challenges associated with a rapidly changing society. The affective as well as the cognitive, psychomotor, and experiential domains of learning are essential components of faculty facilitator preparation.

The American Heritage Dictionary[3] gives several definitions for the word *art*. One of the definitions is, "A specific skill in adept performance, conceived as requiring the exercise of intuitive faculties that cannot be learned solely by study." This definition seems to convey the essence of what is needed to prepare a well rounded faculty facilitator to teach in a nursing program.

Self-Understanding and Awareness

The first aspect of the preparation of the future faculty facilitator is to focus on self-understanding. The faculty facilitator who is self-assured is better able to establish positive faculty facilitator-student interactions. Self-awareness derives from experiences which allow the faculty facilitator to look inward and attempt to flaunt strengths and correct, improve, or de-emphasize weaknesses. There are many techniques used to stimulate self-awareness. One technique is dyadic encounter. In this situation, two people come together and share information about each other. The exchange usually includes the sharing of things that the persons like or dislike about themselves. The process of sharing can be instigated by using a booklet such as *Dyadic Encounter: A Program for Getting Acquainted in Depth*.[4] Each person asks the questions posed in the booklet and listens to the responses. Any question can be answered by a "pass." The questions relate to personal preferences. The questioning takes place in an atmosphere of trust. The listener attempts to be supportive of the person answering the questions. Judgment is withheld. This activity allows the person to hear his/her own answers to the questions which helps to foster self-understanding and awareness. The couple agree to maintain confidentiality. This activity can be repeated at periodic intervals during the faculty facilitator preparation. See also the section on Nurturing Creativity of Nurse as Person (Chapter 9) for other suggestions.

Group Building

The preparation of faculty facilitators includes strategies for encouraging positive group interactions. Many teaching-learning situations take place with students organized in groups. Even large classroom gatherings can be improved by the knowledge of group building techniques. One of the first strategies the faculty facilitator needs to use is a strategy which helps the students to get to know one another. There are numerous ways to achieve this goal. Some exercises follow.

EXERCISES

EXERCISE 1:

Each person is requested to introduce himself/herself and tell one thing about himself, such as: a funny thing that has happened, his/her work, something that stands out about himself, something exciting that recently happened.

The group proceeds in a clockwise direction. The second person will repeat what the first person said (name and fact) and then introduce himself and tell the fact. The next person introduces both previous persons and relates their facts and then adds his name and facts. This continues until the last person names all persons, gives their facts, and adds his/her own name and fact.

EXERCISE 2:

Each person must select another person in the room to interview. He/she should try to interview a person he does not know, or one he knows least about, or one he would like to know more about. Ten minutes is allowed for the interview. Notes should not be taken; the interviewer must trust his/her memory to remember the facts. The first five minutes is devoted to interviewing, then roles can be exchanged so each person interviews the other. At the end of the ten minutes each person should be ready to introduce his/her new friend to the group.

EXERCISE 3:

The group should be split into four subgroups, with each subgroup standing in a circle. Each member should introduce himself/herself and say where he is from. Each person in the circle must repeat the names and places of all the previous persons. When each subgroup completes this activity, the two subgroups can merge together. Then the groups should assemble with every other person standing next to a person from the other group. The same introductory process can then be conducted. Finally the groups merge into the whole group, proceeding with introductions in the same way.

EXERCISE 4:

The names of all the group members are placed in a receptacle (ie, hat, bag, wastepaper basket, etc) which is passed around so each person can pull out a name. Then each person mingles in the group trying to identify the person whose name they have drawn. After each person is identified, the members are introduced to the group by the person who drew their name.

EXERCISE 5:

The trust walk is an opportunity to develop a trust relationship with another person. Each person is assigned a partner who will act as his/her eyes. Once blindfolded, the partner will introduce him to experiences through nonverbal means. The experience is nonverbal. Each person will assume the role of learner for 15 minutes, then the partner will be the learner and he/she will act as his partner's eyes for 15 minutes. After the partners have assumed each role, they will come together and discuss how they felt in each of the roles. Then the whole group is reassembled and asked to discuss the implications of the exercise to the process of group building.

EXERCISE 6:

The group is asked to stand up and start mingling without talking. Then directions are given to group members to greet each person with a variety of greetings: first, a happy eye greeting; next, a sad eye greeting, then a left shoulder tap; then a right shoulder tap; an angry eye greeting; a right hip bump; a left hip bump; and finally a greeting that shows each person that the member is glad he/she is there.

EXERCISE 7:

Sitting in a circle, each person should introduce himself/herself and state a fact which he does not like about himself. Then he/she should state what he likes about himself. After this is completed the group discusses how they felt about the activity and what insights they gained by participating in it.

EXERCISE 8:

Everyone is given a piece of paper and a pencil to write their obituaries in 15 minutes, including all the things they want people to remember about them. After volunteers have read their creations, the implications of the exercise should be discussed. The discussion can be stimulated by asking the group to reflect on what portion of the information they have already achieved as opposed to what they still have to complete to achieve their prophesy. Then, they can try to establish a timetable to meet the goals they established for themselves.

EXERCISE 9:

Persons in the first row and every other row should stand up and turn around. Then the other persons in the hall should stand up. Persons in the odd rows can introduce themselves to persons in the even row, to the person directly in front of them, to the persons on each side of them. Then everyone should be encouraged to greet the persons to the right and left of them in their own row, to wave to a few people that are farthest away from them, to wave to a few people a couple of rows away from them, to throw a kiss or two to someone they'd like to meet later, and then to return to their seats. Everyone should feel free to change seats and sit next to someone else if desired.

EXERCISE 10:

Each person writes a list of nonverbal clues they use in daily interactions. After the list is collected, each set of clues should be read to see if the class can guess who handed in the list. As each person is correctly identified, the group should be asked which clue or clues helped them to identify the person. This helps the students realize the nonverbal clues they use most often.

EXERCISE 11:

After the group has been together awhile, this activity can be tried. The group comes together to identify the strengths of individual members, for example: Carl is excellent in administering CPR; the friendliness of Wanda strengthens the clinical group. Then a list of strengths can be written on a chalkboard. Each member of the group is given an opportunity to select the strength(s) he/she wants to exhibit. After the selection, each person is asked why a particular strength was selected, what will be done with the strength, and how it will change his/her current behavior.

EXERCISE 12:

This exercise is also useful after the group is together awhile. Each person fills in the name of a member of the group that would fill the following roles:

    a student you trust,
    a student to help solve a theory problem,
    a student to help solve a clinical problem,
    a student to share a personal problem with,
    a student that you respect,
    a student that respects you,
    a student that inspires you,
    a student that you enjoy being with,
    a student that helps you with problems,
    a student that irritates you,
    a student that listens to you.

Then the person should look at the list and see how many times he/she selected the same person and determine if it would be possible to increase the numbers of people on his/her list, and why it would be important to do this.

DISCUSSION

Exercises 1 through 12 are designed to help participants get to know one another. The activities attempt to provide repetition and novelty to help participants remember names, know more people, want to know more people, and use verbal and nonverbal forms of communication.

An attempt is made to help the participants understand that they are valued as people. Some of the exercises introduce humor. The humor helps the participants to feel that all of life is not serious—some parts are light and frivolous. The use of exercises to combine the light and frivolous with serious topics of the curriculum is highly recommended.

These exercises are useful in establishing a group, in keeping a group cohesive, or in improving group interactions when the group seems to be having difficulties. Periodic use of group strategies seems to make the group more sensitive to each other's needs and feelings. The competitive nature of some of the educational process tends to put a strain on a group. By interspersing these strategies throughout the semester, the group can be helped to stay together and support one another. The exercises take very little time to complete. The times can be shortened or lengthened depending on the amount of time that is available. The expenditure of time is considered inconsequential when it is compared to the potential benefits that derive from the process.

One word of caution is necessary in relation to groups. MacKinnon[5] notes that some creative persons dislike group activity. His research shows that some creative persons feel stifled by group strategies, preferring to work alone and progress at their own rate outside of the group. If the group is flexible rather than rigid, it is more likely to be acceptable to creative persons.

Teaching Strategies

The creative faculty facilitator is one who is capable of varying teaching strategies to meet the individual learning needs of students. Strategies for achieving individual learning needs include the following:

1) developing learning packages,
2) incorporating a variety of media into instructional designs,
3) using resource persons effectively,
4) structuring time frames in a variety of ways for learning to take place,
5) encouraging self-direction of learners,
6) encouraging students to raise questions,
7) offering a variety of alternatives for meeting objectives,
8) producing a climate of constructive discontent,

9) exhibiting a tolerance for ambiguity,

10) structuring the environment for learning to take place.

The individualized approach to education is conducive to nurturing creative behaviors. This approach allows the learner the flexibility necessary to explore areas of concern and to identify problems which are personally and professionally significant.

During education of educators, opportunities are provided for the learner to participate in teaching-learning situations which develop skill in each of the teaching strategies. The future faculty facilitator is provided opportunities to interact in a teaching role with actual students or with simulated students. Videotaping these sessions allows for a more thorough analysis of the learning situation. The faculty facilitator does not have to be present during the videotaping. However, if the faculty facilitator is present, it is possible to do a teacher-interaction analysis of the future faculty facilitator's performance at the same time it is being videotaped. The teacher-interaction analysis can follow the model of Flanders[6] or Hough and Duncan[7]. This procedure focuses on the teaching strategies and how the future faculty facilitator interacts with the students during the instructional process. This assessment helps to document how the future faculty facilitator spends the majority of time during the teaching/learning period. Examples of ways that faculty facilitators lead groups include giving information, encouraging students to participate in the discussion, clarifying misinformation, giving reinforcement, and so forth. Based on the analysis, it is possible to make prescriptions for changing teaching strategies to encourage students to be active participants in the teaching-learning process. The analysis of the videotape provides the future faculty facilitator with an opportunity to see herself/himself in action. Analysis includes evaluation of the manner of delivery of material, the content and its relevance, and evaluation of the selective media on the basis of production, ease of utilization, ability to emphasize a point, originality, visability, and so forth. The student group can also provide feedback from their perspective about the future faculty facilitator's presentation.

Using simulated students, peers of the future faculty facilitator, is a way to make the feedback very effective. These persons have an excellent knowledge base for evaluating the performance and providing their peer with constructive suggestions. The videotape assessment can focus on the teaching-learning environment and how the future faculty facilitator arranged the environment for learning to take place. Questions can be used to aid the assessment: What changes were made in the environment based on student feedback? Was the future faculty facilitator able to rearrange the teaching strategies based on this feedback? (Note, it is possible to program simulated students to give specific feedback for the future faculty facilitator to respond to.) Assessment of the climate is possible. Did the future faculty facilitator put the students at ease? Did he/she show respect for students? Were students called by name? Were all students included in eye contact at periodic intervals? The future faculty facilitator's handling of questions is also evaluated. How much time did the students have to raise questions? Were their questions dealt with in a satisfactory manner? Did the future faculty facilitator encourage the group to find the answers to their own questions? Were opportunities suggested for future inquiry to take place? Behaviors which suggest an interest in stimulating creative potential are evaluated. During the presentation did the future faculty facilitator use phrases like, "Does anyone else have an idea related to this issue?" "Are there other alternatives?" "Let's brainstorm other possibilities." "Who can think of another way to solve this problem?" "Can someone restate the problem in a creative format?" "Use your imaginations and see if any new ideas occur to you." Did the future faculty facilitator permit productive excursions by the students or did he/she cut off the students prematurely? Was the future faculty facilitator able to decide which excursions were productive and which ones were nonproductive? How did he/she handle nonproductive excursions?

The opportunities the future faculty facilitator builds into the instructional design for encouraging self-direction of students is evaluated during this time. Were there opportunities provided for students to pursue individual interests? Were there a variety of activities incorporated into the instructional design? Were bibliographies and media suggested for encouraging additional inquiry? Were students encouraged to design their own contracts for meeting objectives? Were students who completed a task early encouraged to explore further?

Assignments offered to future faculty facilitators are specific enough to define the parameters for completing objectives but flexible enough to encourage creative endeavors. For example, the criteria for developing learning packages includes the format to be followed (ie, a model such as Herrscher's Individualized Instruction), the latest date the assignment can be accomplished, any things which must be included in the package (ie, examples of media, resources used in production, etc), and the way the activity will be evaluated. Creative aspects of the assignment are encouraged by allowing the future faculty facilitator to select the content to include in the instructional package, to change or use existing media or create new media, and to generate a variety of alternatives for meeting the objectives of the instructional package. The evaluation of the activity is based on an assessment of the creative aspects as well as the identified components. If the creative part of the assignment is not evaluated, the future faculty facilitator may not feel it is as important as the other parts of the assignment. As opposed to letter grades, the grading might be done in the following manner: credit, pass-fail, poor to excellent, or needs improvement.

During the faculty-facilitator preparation it is good to prepare the future faculty member for ways that a traditional educational system can be modified to allow for creativity to survive. Many schools of nursing still rely heavily on the lecture method of presentation. This method is generally considered less conducive to individualized instruction than many other methods of teaching. However, even the large lecture hall can be adapted to creatively involve students in the learning process. One way to achieve this goal is to use as many of the student's senses as possible in the teaching strategy.

Pearson[8] reported an example of how she facilitated the use of five senses of a group of nursing students involved in her research. She combined the eating of a lemon-flavored cup cake with the viewing of a sound film. During the viewing of another film, she sprayed the air with lemon air freshener to provide an experience that combined the use of the five senses: sight, sound, smell, touch and taste. While Pearson was not focusing on unleashing creative potential, her experimental design is an example of the way that the senses can be stimulated to awaken awareness. Hitchhiking on Pearson's ideas, a faculty facilitator is able to stimulate the senses in almost any setting where teaching-learning takes place.

The large lecture hall can be transformed from a hollow area between four walls to an olfactory haven by dispensing small waterproof bags with cotton pledgets soaked with a variety of smells, some pleasing and some displeasing. Parnes[9] uses this methodology with groups of 500 or more. Periodically the participants are directed to stimulate their sense of smell by removing a cotton pledget from the bag. The taste sense can be stimulated in the same way; for example, hard candies can be put in a bag and left at each seat. The tactile sense can be stimulated by placing a variety of different textured materials or articles in the bags. Individualized short assignments can be interspersed throughout the lecture. For example, a student that had a problem calculating a dosage of medication in the clinical laboratory is given a similar short math problem to solve based on a medication associated with the health problem that is being presented in the lecture. While this student is working the math problem, small groups of other students are working on other problems associated with the lecture material.

Transition to Faculty Facilitator

The future faculty facilitator graduates and becomes a faculty member. The autonomy often connected with this role can be rewarding and frightening. The new faculty member frequently does not have a consistent role model or mentor to directly interact with to help encourage the faculty member's development. The new faculty member often finds that academia is a demanding place and the pace is staggering. It is difficult to keep ahead of the students or even to keep up with them. This milieu tends to discourage creativity. In an attempt to keep one's head above water, many of the ideals instilled during graduate school are put aside and survival techniques are instituted. This situation results in both the faculty facilitator and the students losing a great deal from the educational experience. In order for new faculty members to settle in and feel comfortable in their new role, they need to have enough support from their colleagues so they do not feel overwhelmed. The newly prepared faculty member comes with many ideas that are vital to the process of continual rejuvenation of the educational system. These ideas must not wait a year or two to be used. They need to be incorporated immediately. Competent faculty members who feel relatively at ease in the situation must help new faculty members to overcome their reality shock and use their knowledge, skill and empathy to facilitate students through the learning environment.

> *The scholar who cherishes the love of comfort, is not fit to be deemed a scholar.*
>
> Confucius

Loosening-Up Activities

Creative tendencies are an innate capability of all persons. They develop in an environment where people use their imagination, feel free to express new ideas, and appreciate the value of strangeness and diversity. The faculty facilitator who exhibits creative expression encourages students to exhibit this behavior also. Creative expression is likely to emerge if the faculty facilitator spends time "loosening" up the student body. This type of activity is done frequently with preschool and young school-age children, but it is not done often enough with college level students. An exercise such as asking the students to imagine themselves as a dog and scribble off everything that comes to their minds is an example of a "lossening up activity." This exercise allows the student to wander freely without regard for reality or exactness. By including these exercises in classes, the faculty facilitator demonstrates the value of creative thinking and its usefulness in the role development of the professional person.

There are additional "loosening up" exercises that can be utilized. The following examples offer clues for the faculty facilitator to use to vary his/her classes.

EXERCISES

EXERCISE 1:

The facilitator directs the students to take a pack of matches and sit in a circle of eight to ten people. As the match book is passed, each person must take a match, light it, and while it burns tell the group the most exciting professional nursing experience he/she can remember.

If there are several circles of people, after each group completes this task they should decide on the situation they want to share as a group with the other groups. One large circle can be formed and each group can present their chosen situation.

EXERCISE 2:

Each person draws a name tag from a bag. In another bag there should be cards with the following information: numbers of children, years of work experience, age, location of birth, and predictions for future work. Each participant takes five cards from the bag, matches the names and items, and then concocts a short story to present to the group. (ie, Mary Jones, age 42, has worked 15 years, has two children, was born in Lexington, Kentucky, and will be a director of nursing). When you finish reporting the imagined "facts" the person identifies himself/herself and tells how many facts are correct. If he/she feels uncomfortable, he can correct the incorrect facts.

EXERCISE 3:

Students follow the directions on a record, such as "Get Fit While You Sit." (This is a record on movements and people delight in doing the simple exercises.)

EXERCISE 4:

Listening to a creative movement record, each person closes his/her eyes and lets the music take him to a far away place. As the music plays, the faculty facilitator begins a narrative: they are in a boat; there is something on the horizon; it is getting closer; the boat continues to speed ahead. The narrative ends there and the group is encouraged to finish their fantasy to the sound of the music. Once the music ends, the group is asked to share their stories.

EXERCISE 5:

After watching a short film, such as the "Dot and the Line" or "Pack Your Own Chute," the group has a free discussion of the ideas that the film triggered in their minds.

EXERCISE 6:

After the class is paired off, the partners sit back to back. One person is given a slip of paper with a design on it, and he/she must give directions to his partner, who has a plain piece of paper and a pencil. As the directions are given, the partner draws the diagram without asking any questions. Then the roles are reversed. After both partners have completed both roles, they share and compare the original diagrams with the drawn ones. Then they discuss how they felt in the roles.

DISCUSSION

Exercises 1 through 6 are examples of exercises that can be interspersed in any course or in faculty meetings. They are easy to implement and can be done in almost any setting. Minor adaptations in the exercises increase their usability.

Student Assignments

The success or failure of creative assignments is closely associated with how effectively the faculty facilitator is able to communicate the goals of the experience. Just as the student is influenced by many feelings, so too is the faculty facilitator. It is hypothesized that how the faculty facilitator feels about self, about associates, and about the environment that surrounds him/her will play a part in the way the faculty facilitator role is enacted. Attitudes and beliefs of the faculty facilitator play a part in how information is communicated and exchanged with students. A creative assignment can be asphyxiated by a faculty facilitator who lacks the enthusiasm to teach and lacks the ability to guide students in the process of discovery.

The faculty facilitator and students collaborate on the assignments for the course. Some assignments are more faculty-directed while some are student-directed. In either case, the creative component of the assignment is stressed. For example, a faculty objective might relate to knowing the basic four food groups. The student decides how to meet the objective. The objective can be met by writing a paper, buying food in a store which represents each of the four groups, making a poster, doing an audio tape on the basic four foods, and so forth. The flexibility provided by a broader objective allows the student to be more creative about how to meet the objective.

Student creativity can be nurtured through feedback on assignments. Students usually spend a great deal of time thinking about the information they include in required papers or other written assignments. This thinking process is part of creative problem solving. The student cannot remember indefinitely what thought processes went into reaching the conclusions that were expressed. Therefore, the faculty facilitator needs to provide thoughtful feedback to the students as soon as possible. It is possible for the student to be asked to discuss how a particular conclusion was reached. In recapturing the thought process, the student can discover inconsistencies or errors in thinking. This type of evaluation is much more valuable than assigning grades or correcting papers with red pencils. This evaluation process encourages the student to continue in the problem solving framework even after the specific assignment is completed. This approach encourages continuous learning as opposed to fragmented learning divided by assignments and grades. Following this alternative design, assignments become stepping stones to new and valuable learning.

Creative, Affective, and Critical Thinking

The faculty facilitator who encourages creative potential in students must be able to combine creative, affective, and critical elements in the right portions in the curriculum. The model which guides this process is first— WIDE, DIVERGENT, FREE-FLOWING, and CREATIVE—then—NARROW, CONVERGENT, ANALYTIC, and CRITICAL.[10]

Much of the criticism of creative problem-solving techniques arise from the perception that there is a heavy emphasis on the first stage of the model and too little emphasis placed on the second stage. Actually, these criticisms are unjustified if the creative problem-solving process is utilized correctly. The faculty facilitator provides opportunities for both of these stages to develop. The "loosening up" exercises are examples of exercises that relate to the first stage of the model with very little attention being given to the second stage. If they are viewed as an isolated activity, rather than as part of the total educational experience, they could be judged as focusing on only the lighter part of the process. However, when they are viewed as part of the total educational process they are placed in their proper perspective. Other parts of the educational experience are mostly critical in nature and counterbalance the early emphasis placed on the creative loosening up activities.

The faculty facilitator's role is to facilitate and manage learning. The faculty facilitator sows the seeds for students to grow. In this teaching role, the title of faculty facilitator is most appropriate. The learning environment serves as a vehicle for developing awareness in students. Awareness escalates by paying attention to details. Activities that develop the student's awareness follow.

EXERCISES

EXERCISE 1:

The students go to a hospital unit for an hour to observe the environment. They are asked to pay special attention to details and to use all their senses in the observation.

After they have observed and returned, they are given a large white sheet of paper and colored pencils or magic markers to draw what they saw, complete with descriptive labels.

Two or three students should explain their drawings. Then time should be allowed for all the students to make changes based on the discussion. The students return to the hospital and compare their drawings with what they observed while there. They can make changes in the drawings at this time also. Once they are back with the group again they all can discuss what they missed, misinterpreted, changed, or added, and finally what they learned from the activity.

EXERCISE 2:

The group observes the room in detail for five minutes and then close their eyes. Individuals are called on to identify the location of objects in the room; one student acts as monitor and records the location of the identified object and where the student located it (ie, "Mary, Where is the eraser?" Monitor records the eraser is on the right hand corner of the ledge on the front chalk board. Response: the eraser is on the teacher's desk).

After a number of objects are identified, the monitor reads off the list. The participants can explain how they decided on their answers and how they felt about responding. The group is encouraged to pay more attention to details in their everyday surroundings.

EXERCISE 3:

One frame of a filmstrip is shown and then turned off. Students are asked to write down all the details they observed in the scene. The scene is shown on the screen again and compared with the students' lists. They then discuss what details were omitted and why certain details were omitted. The numbers of omissions or errors in the list are counted. After showing a second frame and completing the same process, the students can see if there is improvement in observation skills.

EXERCISE 4:

Using a room with a one-way viewing window, the students observe a client situation while it is being videotaped concurrently. The videotape is shown while a student gives the description of the observation to the class, then the video is rerun so the student can observe it. The accuracy of the observations and reporting can be discussed with the following questions: Were the discrepancies potentially dangerous? Were the omissions important? Did the reporting give a clear picture of what took place?

EXERCISE 5:

The students write a synopsis of their best nursing care given this week. When the class seems to be slowing down, the faculty facilitative introduces a short passage of music. After a short period he/she sprays the room with a scent such as lemon, pine, or coconut. Then he/she changes the light-darkness factor in the room. After a few more minutes the students are asked to discuss the vingettes and what influence the stimulation of senses had on their productivity. Then they should describe the poorest nursing intervention they did recently and they should deliberately assess how they could improve it paying special attention to environmental factors.

DISCUSSION

Exercises 1 through 5 are deliberate attempts to improve the observation skills of students. So much of the environment is taken for granted that exercises are needed to focus attention on details. In the nursing profession, observation must be a highly perfected skill. Exercises like these can be repeated and repeated until observations become extremely keen and nothing is taken for granted.

Never take anything for granted.

Benjamin Disraeli

Assessing the Environment

The hospital provides a rich resource for assessing the effects of the environment on the client's ability to recover from illness. The objectives of the experience stress the use of all the senses for completing the evaluation. Brainstorming and deferred judgment are used to generate hypotheses on how to improve the environment to help the client to restore his/her health whenever it is a feasible goal.

The faculty facilitator plans the sessions with groups of five to seven students. They tour the facilities, stopping to observe key locations. The observations focus on odors, colors, textures, clutter, storage, seating arrangements, interactions with clients, accessibility to toilet facilities, food, telephones, and so forth. The students are encouraged to identify all the positive things they observe as well as all the negative things. When negative things are identified, they brainstorm ways to improve the situation as illustrated in the following examples.

EXAMPLES

EXAMPLE 1:

On a pediatric unit, the students noted that the walls were painted drab colors which the children did not like. Brainstorming ways to improve the situation, they developed a list of potential ideas for transforming the barren walls into child-centered walls. They suggested placing children's art work at eye level, putting up pictures the children draw themselves, putting up bulletin boards to decorate, hanging chalk boards, placing large sheets of plain newsprint and giving the children magic markers, advertising for an art class to come in and paint murals, having a contest and rewarding the child who comes up with the most creative idea, decorating with posters, asking the art museum to bring paintings which can be changed periodically, or wallpapering one wall with paper designed for children.

EXAMPLE 2:

In an unoccupied room, students are blindfolded and asked to try to imagine and experience how they can get their belongings, get to the bathroom, call the nurse, and telephone their family in this unfamiliar setting.

After several students experience this situation, they discuss how it feels to be a client with limited visual ability or in a dark unfamiliar room. They then brainstorm ways to make the environment more conducive to the needs of clients. This exercise usually emphasizes the importance for lowering beds, having call lights within reach, placing telephones in accessible areas, having light switches outside bathroom doors, and having furnishings and equipment out of the traffic pattern within rooms.

EXAMPLE 3:

The students are blindfolded and sit on chairs in the main hall of one of the in-patient units. They focus their attention on auditory observations. It heightens their awareness of the noise that interferes with rest and recovery of clients. The sounds they note are paging systems, ringing telephones, objects falling on the floor, elevator doors opening and closing, professionals discussing "cases," persons asking directions, voices summoning other persons, laughter, televisions with a variety of programs, coughing, IPPB equipment, rattle of dishes, clanging of test tubes, wheels rumbling on the linoleum, and an occasional moan.

After the blindfolds are removed, the students' discussion brings out that the noises are frightening when you cannot see them. They note that most clients are not able to see what is going on from their rooms so the sounds probably are interpreted by them in the same way. They also note that the hospital is not a restful place. Most of the time there is some noise. Short periods of quiet are interrupted by bursts of unpleasant sounds. Unpleasant or unfamiliar sounds are far more prevalent than pleasant sounds. They conclude that attention must be focused on controlling noise if clients are going to receive enough rest to help them recover in the least amount of time.

This exercise should be repeated at various times of the day in order to compare the noise levels and to emphasize the increasing importance of diminishing the noise as nighttime appears.

EXAMPLE 4:

The students are asked to close their eyes and run their fingers over various areas that the client comes in contact with. They focus on the sheets, seats and arms of chairs, hospital clothing, surfaces of treatment tables, seats and arms of wheelchairs, and surfaces of stretchers. Special attention is placed on the temperature of these areas. It is found that many surfaces are cold to touch and many feel coarse and displeasing. A few are soft and warm. A comparison is made of the surfaces that the clients spend the majority of time in contact with and with the areas that they contact less frequently. The bed linens are identified as high contact areas and are categorized as coarse and displeasing. The effects of contacts with displeasing surfaces are identified as a source of potential client dissatisfaction.

EXAMPLE 5:

Students are required to eat a hospital meal paying special attention to hot and cold, texture, aesthetic qualities, choices, spicing, amounts, and ease of eating. The discussion following the meal brings out that the students do not agree on many things related to the food. This helps to highlight that clients have similar diverse reactions to food. The students acknowledge that one client can find fault with the same offering that another client finds enjoyable. Furthermore, emphasizing the use of the taste sense heightens the student's awareness of the importance of food to the recovery of clients as well as to the clients who are in the hospital for evaluation. They note that when food becomes one of the major activities of the day, it takes on added importance.

Faculty Responsibilities— A Creative Approach

The faculty member quickly learns that facilitating learning is only part of the responsibilities that are assumed when accepting a position on a faculty. The faculty member assumes responsibility for participating in committee work, contributing to the university or college at large, contributing to the community, participating in professional organizations, and demonstrating scholarly writing and research. These requirements of the position are certain to require the use of creativity to be accomplished effectively. It sometimes takes creativity just to survive in the system as the demands seem overwhelming to the novice faculty member who is struggling to be the best educator that is possible.

It may be necessary to select areas on which to concentrate efforts rather than trying to respond to all the requirements at one time. The faculty member needs to negotiate a contract with a decision-maker clearly identifying where he/she will concentrate his creative talents. For instance, writing allows for more creative expression than research, therefore, writing is a better choice for the creative faculty facilitator. The faculty member bases the choices on personal preference as well as overall faculty needs. For instance, if the nursing faculty needs representation on university committees, the faculty member is entitled to evaluate the charge of the committee and see if his/her creative talent can be utilized effectively on the committee. If the committee's goals are inconsistent with the faculty member's talents, the committee would probably be better served through participation of another faculty member. Unfortunately, this type of selection is not always possible but the design might lead to more satisfaction in faculties as well as more productive committees.

Writing is an excellent medium for expressing creativity. The way that ideas can be communicated in written form is almost limitless. The faculty member can write letters to the editor, short articles for circulars, articles for journals or newspapers, chapters in books, books, poems, hints for sharing columns, articles for lay magazines, health education pamphlets, critiques of other's work, and so forth. The stimulus to write can be increased by doing exercises like the ones found on page 72.

The faculty member who makes writing an obligation often improves his/her teaching ability as writing requires a clear communication of ideas, and this is excellent practice for improving other means of communication. In addition, writing requires the faculty member to review the literature related to the selected topic, and this results in the latest ideas being included in teaching-learning situations.

Community contributions frequently offer opportunities for faculty members to express their creativity. The community has so many needs that creativity can be expressed by creating new services to meet community needs or by participation in services already available. For instance, creating a nursing clinic in an underserved area is an outstanding achievement and a viable alternative in some communities. In another area, the faculty member might add an additional service in an already existing service. An example is offering human sexuality seminars in an elementary school. In another situation, the faculty member might be able to participate creatively in the situation as it currently exists. For example, a faculty member participates as a volunteer in the Reach for Recovery program. Although there is an established format which is extremely effective, she expresses her creativity by offering ideas for improving the training of additional volunteers.

The faculty member who values the expression of creativity can find many opportunities to derive satisfaction. The clue is for the faculty member to look at the situation as a challenge which can bring satisfaction. Rather than being overwhelmed by the challenge, the creative individual breaks down the whole into small manageable parts which respond to creative attack. The challenge is great but the rewards for success are greater!

Another way for the faculty member to increase creativity is to deliberately study the behaviors of faculty colleagues that are creative. It is good to try to understand how creative people differ from less creative people and to attempt to simulate creative behaviors. Creative persons use their time differently, and studying how they go about being creative helps others understand how to improve their personal skills in this area. An assumption is made here that creative people are more productive, and productivity is essential if a faculty member is to survive in the system. Additionally, to learn more about how creative persons in other disciplines use their time, the faculty member can be enriched by studying the lifestyles of artists, composers, dancers, playwrights, dramatists, sculptors, writers, poets, architects, musicians, and inventors.

Many people who are eager to express their creativity find it necessary to have space available, away from their desks and offices, to achieve their goal. This creative space is more conducive to thinking than is the traditional space allotted to faculty members on the basis of so many square feet per person. Even some nursery schools have allotted "time out space" for children, realizing that getting away from the ordinary activities of the day can be a beautiful thing. In this creative space, it is possible for persons to be alone and engage in whatever activity they find valuable for renewal, such as a nap, jogging, sitting and staring into space, listening to music, meditating, or whatever.

Some creative persons feel that getting outside the building is more conducive to creative expression. For these faculty members, a short walk or run where they can commune with nature facilitates their creative expression. During the outside caper, special attention is paid to everything. Every creature, happening, and work of nature receives special attention allowing the faculty member to use the experiences to help solve problems back at the office or in the clinical setting. The interlude from the actual work of the day is often successful in breathing new life into the situation which helps in the problem-solving process.

A word of caution is necessary here. The faculty member who is interested in being creative needs to seek out an organization that is ready to accept this model as a viable alternative to more traditional models. One example that an organization allows creative activities is found in the way time is structured. A faculty member cannot be overburdened with student contact and committee requirements and still have sufficient time to be creative. At least one organization has allotted 10% of the employee's time free "to play around with ideas, explore things." Included in the formula for producing creative ideas was an allocation of time to get *information*—not a lecture or instructions—but information."

While there are no clear-cut prescriptions for generating and nurturing creativity in faculty members, research now strongly supports that practicing some of the suggestions found throughout this book will climax in more creative persons. Unfortunately, one of the major detriments to faculty members increasing their creative potential is their own hesitancy to do so. Faculty members, whose colleagues reward logical thinking, sometimes are reluctant to expose their preference for creative thinking. Fortunately, creative thinking is beginning to receive greater acclaim and will eventually assume equal status with logical thinking. At that point, more faculty members will be rewarded for creativity and be eager to let everyone know they possess it.

> *The man who never alters his opinions is like standing water,*
> *and breeds reptiles of the mind.*
>
> William Blake

Conclusion

The faculty facilitator is one of the key actors in the educational process. The preparation of faculty facilitators is an essential responsibility of every profession. The preparation needs to provide a broad base of knowledge, understanding, and experiences so the graduate of the program is adequately prepared to function in a system that is continually changing. Opportunities are provided to use critical, analytical, and creative thinking to stimulate right and left hemisphere brain potential.

The faculties of schools of nursing need to focus attention on nurturing the creative potential of their members. The responsibilities assumed by faculty members provide a wide range of ways to use creative potential effectively. Faculty members will benefit personally and professionally through their use of creative potential. Most importantly, the clients and the nursing professional will also benefit by nursing faculty increasing their creative as well as their logical thinking abilities.

Chapter 11

Nurturing Creativity in Students of Nursing

Many of the ideas presented in the section on nurturing creativity in faculty facilitators are equally relevant to this section. Creative faculty facilitators are to the students as the yolk of the egg is to the white of the egg. Both are vital components—one to the egg and the other to the teaching-learning process. Therefore, it is not unexpected that ideas relating to nurturing creativity in faculty facilitators should relate to nurturing creativity in students as well.

At the risk of sounding too simplistic, the assumption is made that a school of nursing known as a good place to work and study is very likely to offer a successful educational program.

The potentiality that the nursing profession will endure is closely associated with the quality and quantity of the students that elect to study the discipline. The students currently selecting nursing represent a variety of backgrounds. They fall into a wider range of ages than previously; they have a diversity of intellectual endowment; and they come from a variety of socioeconomic backgrounds. There are an increasing number of males and individuals from various ethnic groups represented in student population, but these groups are still below the numbers reflecting their existence in the population at large. The heterogenity of the student body makes it necessary to individualize instruction in order that each student is given the opportunity to reach his/her maximum potential.

Moustakas[1] wisely counsels that a person's potential and promise are reflected in his/her desire for additional experiences rather than in his/her past records, scores, or grades. The best way to know a person is to view him/her in relation to his own interests, desires, and experiences.

Broudy[2] proposes an analogy, if not taken too literally, that perceiving an interesting personality has some of the identical qualities perceived in works of art. Although Broudy makes the statement with caution, there seems to be a correlation between personal and artistic creations that is difficult to dispute from experience. Persons with interesting personalities frequently bring joy to the perceiver. The joy is significant enough to warrant the nurturance of personality traits or artistic creations as valued components of society which are achievable through the educational process.

Climates for Creativity

Goodland[3] traces the evolution of the goals of educational programs. He notes that it was not until the twentieth century that the goal of education was expanded to include the goals of personal or self-realization. He suggests that these goals include a wide range of skills related to knowledge, values, sciences, the humanities, and aesthetic sources of human enlightenment. The inclusion of skills related to these areas in early educational programs should eventually result in students entering college with a broader base of experience than was previously the case.

The human environment that provides love, safety, belonging, acceptance, and respect for people has the basic conditions for growth to take place. Under these conditions, the student is provided the arena for self-actualization of his/her potential. The faculty facilitator nurtures the situation by offering resources, making opportunities available, giving helpful information when it is needed or sought, and by being available to students. Providing a nonthreatening atmosphere for learning to take place results in the student being more spontaneous and open and consequently more creative. While the student assumes the responsibility for his/her own learning, the situation which fosters this learning is structured to limit threats to self, to respect the uniqueness of individuals, and to allow the learner the freedom to explore in the light of his/her own interests, desires, and potentialities.

An assumption is made in this volume that the nurturance of the *imagination* is an integral and essential part of the educational process. There is no attempt made to gloss over this assumption as skills in the use of imagination are qualitatively just as important as skills in knowledge acquisition. Unfortunately, there has been a period in our educational history when skills related to the nurturance of the imagination were considered unworthy of consideration and held suspect by nonbelievers. The suspicion surrounding the use of imagination is fortunately beginning to decrease, and educators can openly admit that they are engaged in nurturing the imagination of students. Broudy[2] makes an excellent point when he stresses that concepts, logically and psychologically, come later than percepts. Percepts are images. Image making and image perceiving are imagination. Therefore, imagination cannot be left unattended to in the educational process while cognitive and problem-solving skills receive concentrated effort. To be successful in cognitive and problem-solving endeavors, attention must be focused on the relationship between the imagination and other functions of the mind. Therefore, imagination is a required component of the educational process.

Students should be encouraged to read while using the imagination.

Reading print to merely gain cognitive skills is like eating to only gain nutrition. The student who uses imagination to transform the knowledge into workable solutions to problems will gain much more from reading assignments. Reading, with awareness, is an exciting experience and stimulates the student to dig into the material to make it useful and relevant to other learning which is taking place. For example, the student who reads about the use of play with hospitalized children while using his/her imagination to determine how to integrate this information for the child client in the hospital will expand the knowledge base farther than the student who just reads to complete the assignment. The use of the imagination allows the written word to be transformed into useful ideas to meet the current needs of the student who is attempting to learn about the hospitalized child and his/her needs. Reading, combined with imagination, takes longer than reading for purely cognitive achievement, but it is more useful. As Broudy[2] points out, students who have impoverished imagination stores do not really read, they simply undergo a process of decoding mechanical images.

While curriculums are supposed to include competency in relation to self-realization, there is one fallacy connected with this assumption. There is reason to believe that the educational system may not be able to deliver in the area of personal or self-realization. Goodland[3] suggests that in order to achieve this goal it is necessary to redirect learning to include enriched opportunities to derive a variety of meanings and to devise creative individual approaches to understanding and to problem solving. The commitment to structure educational efforts in this direction may be lacking. A climate which supports the expression of creativity is characterized by the following: a) freedom to explore new ways of doing, b) support provided for trying new ideas, c) individuals rewarded for their efforts, d) individuals trusted to complete objectives, e) punishment and ridicule for making mistakes withheld, f) a high level of morale evident in the setting, and g) a determination to encourage people to keep trying even when problems seem insurmountable.

A climate with these characteristics is not consistently found in institutions that prepare nursing professionals. This situation can be partially explained on the basis of the historical evolution of the profession. Evolving from hospital based vocational training to professional preparation in universities has been a costly proposition for the profession in terms of time, attitudes, and finances. Many of the early hospital programs discouraged creative expression and supported a posture of unquestioning obedience to the medical profession. The scars left from this developmental period are still visible today. Some nurses still tend to fear the independent role and to deaden their creative potential by being dependent on others. These attitudes of practicing nurses are modeled for students of nursing. Students readily adopt the behaviors of role models who they perceive to be successful in their chosen profession.

Another reason that climates that are conducive to nurturing creative potential are not common in nursing may relate to the life-death arena in which clinical practice is studied. The student is impressed, at an early stage in the educational process, with the importance of nursing actions to the survival of clients. Nursing errors are costly to clients and can also be costly to the other health professionals responsible for the client's care. The crisis-oriented setting of a hospital seems to demand one-answer solutions to problems, the *right* answer. The hospital setting seems to demand quick solutions to problems based on facts and precedence rather than on creative solutions that are untried. In addition, learning must take place very quickly. The student needs to learn a great deal in a very short period of time. The 12 week quarter or the 15 week semester becomes the criteria for assessing success or failure. Within this framework, the student becomes accustomed to learning only what is essential to pass examinations and other evaluative methodologies in order to remain in the program. The expression of creative potential is suppressed in order to survive in the system. Moustakas[4] stresses the point that creative energy is stifled when it is restricted. When creative energy is stifled, the spontaneous sense of direction is lost, the sense of being dies, and the creative urge is lost. This situation is a costly one for the profession as creativity is essential to self-renewal of the profession as well as to self-renewal of individuals.

In a recent exchange with a faculty member, the following statement was made, "I think it is important to have every faculty member doing it exactly the same way. The students are confused by the varied requirements expected by faculty." In reply to that statement, the suggestion was made that perhaps we do students a favor exposing them to a variety of ways to achieve goals. We need to help students be able to deal with ambiguity, to face failure and frustration while at the same time allowing them the freedom to create new solutions to problems. Students who develop a tolerance for ambiguity are better prepared to face real world situations which are filled with ambiguity and conducted by a diverse group of individuals.

Characteristics of Creative Students

The creative student prefers to have few limits placed on his/her activities. Based on MacKinnon's[5] research as faculty facilitators trying to nurture creative potential of students, we need to use caution in setting stringent limits on those being nurtured. This hypothesis is based on the realization that the creative person is open to responding to experiences from within and without. Limitations place restrictions on one's ability to respond and consequently impinge on one's ability to be creative. The characteristics of self-control, coupled with self-discipline, are enough to provide direction for the creative person to learn.

Adequate intelligence is essential for solving problems creatively. However, it is established that having a higher intellectual endowment does not necessarily predispose a person to greater creative ability. In other words, adequate intelligence is a prerequisite to creative behavior but having higher intelligence does not guarantee that a greater creative potential exists. The way that the person choses to utilize intelligence is what matters when considering creativity.

> *It is not the brains that matter most, but that which guides them—the character, the heart, generous qualities, progressive ideas.*
>
> Fyostor Dostoyevski

Creative students are willing to come at a problem from a variety of directions, being relatively assured that attempts at problem solving will be successful if they perservere long enough. Creative students are risk-takers because they do not fear failing on their first attempt, they merely try again using a new approach. This determination usually pays off, and the creative student reaps the benefits of what might seem to be disorganized behavior to more traditional faculty facilitators or to nurses who tend to reward students for finding one solution to a problem in the least amount of time.

> *Fear of ideas makes us impotent and ineffective.*
> Stephen A. Douglas

The creative student has some characteristics which are indistinguishable from their less creative counterparts. Actually, the creative student does not stand out in a crowd, but over a period of time the creative student is likely to achieve at a higher level of excellence.

Now then, what happens when the role of the faculty facilitator necessitates correcting a student? Does this situation result in a lowering of the student's self-esteem and decrease the potential for creativity? When the faculty facilitator continues to show an interest in the student and tries to understand his/her feelings and wishes, a lowering of self-esteem is not likely to occur. The student-faculty facilitator relationship is strengthened through interactions which reflect a consideration of the value of each as a person. The stronger the established bond, the more likely the student is able to maintain his/her integrity and grow rather than be traumatized by constructive criticism or corrective feedback.

Attitudes Associated with Creativity

Students are often heard making statements such as, "I can't do it" or "With my luck it won't happen." Statements like these tend to interfere with student success in educational programs. The former statement reflects a defeatist attitude towards learning as well as being a self-depreciating statement. The latter statement insinuates that the student's luck is worse than other's luck and blames the lack of success on this situation. The statement reflects an attitude of negativism. Neither of these statements are reflective of attitudes compatible with creative behaviors. The former statement, transformed into a creative statement, would read, "In what ways might I succeed?" or "How might I do it successfully?" The restatment of the intent reflects a more positive attitude and a willingness to try to resolve the problem rather than drawing the premature conclusion that success is not possible. The latter statement is probably more serious to resolve as it reflects a negative feeling state about self that needs to be explored in order to get at the real reason that the student believes that his/her luck is any worse than anyone else's. Statements like the two presented are indicators that students need guidance to develop more positive attitudes about self and about learning.

The student who maintains the attitude that learning is possible and that each new situation is a challenge worth his/her attention is able to use creative talent and enjoy learning. Attitudes tend to influence the student's willingness to become involved in and to stay involved with the educational process. If the student is able to retain the attitude that learning is possible, it makes it more likely that he/she will approach each new experience with anticipation and self-confidence and use creativity freely.

Students who have the attitude that they will fail are less likely to use their creative potential to solve problems. Instead, these students try to find the "right answer" to overcome their fear of failing and thus fulfill their prophesy of failure. It is difficult to be excited about learning in the face of anticipated failure or rejection.

Some attitudes are very firmly ingrained in students. The student who has the attitude that learning is not fun or that learning cannot be achieved needs more help to be able to use creative potential effectively. Most of the exercises in this book can be used to help the student to get over the attitudes which interfere with their desire to explore extensively and be successful in an educational setting.

Process Education

The emphasis of educational programs is on *process* rather than subject *content.* The emphasis on process is selected because it usually results in a greater understanding of the whole. It is possible, when the emphasis is placed on content, to know facts and not be able to see relationships between the isolated facts and the whole. An emphasis on facts or content, rather than on process, interferes with the student's opportunity to create new relationships. Or as aptly noted by Heintz, Fieweger, and Fitzgerald[6], the student's knowledge can grow but the student fails to mature unless the educational encounter emphasizes process as opposed to content. They note further that knowledge may help students understand their own emotions but a knowledge base is not sufficient for making them a sensitive person. In the nursing profession, it is imperative that students develop the sensitivity essential for providing humanistic care to the clients they serve.

> *Get your facts first, and then you can distort them as much as you please.*
>
> Mark Twain

Rosen[7] proposes the following statement which exemplifies the importance of process or contrasts the "what we do" with the "what we should do." He suggests that a human...

> ...has a biologically rooted needed to engage in complex activities. ...And it is the activities themselves which are (essential), not the ends which are supposed to be attained by them; these ends are the inessentials and the by-products. Somehow, we have gotten turned around so as to believe that, on the contrary, the ends are primary and the means secondary.[7]

What does all this mean and why is it important? In a rapidly changing, technological society, people are faced with coping with a great number of new situations in a relatively short period of time. We must learn to cope effectively with these changes. The learning process necessary in these changing times includes being capable of creative thinking, being able to relate on a feeling level, being able to clarify values, and being capable of critical thinking. These capabilities help people cope and keep up with the changes they face. The identified capabilities are usually present in persons who feel good about themselves. Therefore, it is a goal of the educational process to provide learning experiences which help the students to gain self-worth so they will be prepared to cope successfully.

The student has to feel a need to learn. When he/she feels this need, motivation is aroused to satisfy the need. The student is encouraged to describe a plan of action, the methodology to carry out the plan of action, and a time frame in which to complete the learning task. A key consideration when developing the plan is to be certain that the plan includes an emphasis on the creative as well as the critical, affective, and psychomotor aspects of learning.

A way to achieve this is illustrated in the following example.

EXAMPLE

Mary feels the need to complete a project to know more about the care of children with cystic fibrosis. Joan feels the need to complete a project to know more about the care of children who are abused. They agree to be a team. They decide to brainstorm ideas for their projects. The following lists emerged from the brainstorming session.

Mary (cystic fibrosis)

dietary control
medications for
respiratory treatment of
emotional reaction to
special school consider-
    ations
implications on the family
financial resources for
hereditary aspects of
incidence of
complications of
opportunities for social
    interaction
special books for
hospitalization of
history of
review of literature in
    relation to
health education for child
health education for com-
    munity
care of child with

special games for
 What makes things complicated
    for these children?
What makes things complicated
    for their parents?
What makes things complicated
    for the professionals caring
    for them?
learning to live with
research related to
nursing's role in relation to
ideal home environment for
school opportunities for
ideal school opportunities for
need for playmates
need for empathy
frustration resulting from

Joan (child abuse)

incidence of
ages of
parents of
groups for abusive parents
emergency networks
funding for
child care programs for
group rehabilitation of parents

research related to
What makes things compli-
cated for these children?
What makes things compli-
cated for their parents?
What makes things compli-
cated for the professionals
caring for them?

interdisciplinary approach to
review of literature of
community resources for
films related to
health education for community
exploration of family with
  history of
emotional make-up of
  abusive parents
emotional responses of
  abused children
re-establishing self-worth
  of abusive parents
promoting self-esteem of
fears of parents who abuse
fear of
building buddy system for
building buddy system for
  abusive parents
frustrations of

nursing's role in relation to
ideal home environment for
effects of the moon on the
  parent's behavior
effects of pollutants on the
  parents' behavior
need for affection
frustration of parents

The two lists contain similarities. Mary and Joan decide that, even though there are common concerns for both groups of children, they will pursue individual projects.

Now they use critical analysis in their deliberations. They look at one list at a time and determine ideas that fit into like categories. The categories they form follow:

Mary (cystic fibrosis)

Treatment modalities

—dietary control
—medications for
—respiratory treatment of

Epidemiology

—hereditary aspects of
—incidence of
—complications of
—history of
—research related to
—review of literature related to

Feeling/Emotional Aspects

—emotional reactions to
—need for playmates
—need for empathy
—frustrations resulting from
—implications on the family
—learning to live with
—opportunities for social interaction

Environmental Projects

—special school considerations
—what makes things complicated for these children?
—what makes things complicated for their parents?
—what makes things complicated for the professionals caring for them?
—ideal home environment for
—school opportunities for
—ideal school opportunities for

Learning Opportunities Projects

—special games for
—special books for

Professional Activities Related to

—financing resources for
—hospitalization of
—health education for child
—health education for family
—health education for community
—care of child with
—nursing's role in relation to

Joan (child abuse)

Environmental Projects

—parents of
—groups for abusive parents
—emergency networks
—group rehabilitation of parents
—child care programs for
—community resources for
—building buddy system for
—building buddy system for abusive parents
—what makes things complicated for these children?

—what makes things complicated for their parents?
—what makes things complicated for the professionals caring for them?
—ideal home environment for

Feeling/Emotional Projects

—exploration of family with history
—emotional make-up of abusive parents
—emotional responses of abused children
—re-establishing self-worth of abusive parents
—promoting self-esteem of
—fears of parents who abuse
—effects of the moon on the parents' behavior
—effects of pollutants on the parents' behavior
—need for affection
—frustrations of
—frustrations of parents

Epidemiology of

—research related to
—ages of
—incidence of
—review of literature of

Professional Activities Related to

—health education for community
—interdisciplinary approach to
—nursing's role in relation to
—funding of

Learning Opportunities Projects

—films related to

You will note that the categories are broad. In addition, they are not constricting. Items can be moved from one category to another based on the student's perception of the item.

The lists can be analyzed in yet another way. Mary and Joan analyze the ideas and decide if they involve mostly critical thinking, creative thinking, feelings and values (affective), or combinations of these. Then they decide what idea lends itself to the type project they really wish to complete. Each student selected a project that involved each aspect of the creative process so they chose the following:

Mary—Frustrations resulting from cystic fibrosis
Joan—Building a buddy system for children who are abused

The next step was to look at the selected topic and Joan asked the following questions of Mary (then Mary asked Joan the same questions).

 1) Why does this topic appeal to you?
 2) What do you like about it?
 3) What do you dislike about it?
 4) What resources will you need to complete the project?
 5) Do you have the time to complete the project?
 6) Who can you get to help with the project?
 7) Are there obstacles to completing your goal?
 8) How will you evaluate your project?
 9) Where will you go for resources?
10) When will you get started?

The use of the questions is an example of a divergent-convergent process. It forces the student to critically analyze the implications of the selected choice. Based on the answers given to the questions the interrogator may try to convince the partner to change, alter, or pursue the project as selected.

Student projects that evolve from a combination of creative and critical analysis tend to differ from projects that evolve from purely critical analysis. Given an assignment, by critical analysis, a student often jumps at the first idea that comes to mind and begins to explore it immediately. The subject is not always of high interest and the enthusiasm for the task easily wanes, whereas projects selected on the basis of creative as well as critical analysis seem to hold the student's attention longer and establish a climate for discovery to take place.

There are frequent notations in the literature about the creativity expressed by the child. One needs only to observe the child, especially the toddler and preschooler, to be convinced of the truth of these statements. White[8] notes that knowledge is a function of being. He suggests that when there is a change in the *being* there is a corresponding change in the knowledge level of the individual. Therefore, as a child grows he/she becomes more knowledgeable. However, the increase in knowledge allows the child to base actions on acceptable established practices which in turn decreases his/her use of spontaneity and intuitive actions. This change in behavior is the hypothesized reason that children grow less creative with increasing years. They become less dependent on the process of discovery when they develop a large data base of knowledge which they systematically use to solve the problems they face. In essence, they allow their intuitive capabilities to deteriorate through underutilization. The deterioration of the ways that young children discover their world is unfortunate as it is apparent that children enjoy learning by discovery, and they actually learn a great deal through this methodology. The young child produces many creative products that are valuable if viewed within the perspective of the child's world rather than from the perspective of the adult's world. If the child continues to use intuition in combination with increasing knowledge base, his/her creative products have the potential for greatness. Somehow, we need to be certain that, as there is a change in the being of the knower, there is a corresponding positive change in the intuitive power of the individual, as well. Otherwise, we will always be in the position of trying to recapture the creative potential of children after it is lost rather than nurturing it from its inception.

Discovery is an essential concept related to the quest for creativity. Discovery takes time to complete. Its purpose is to involve the individual in a situation which allows the free exploration or guided exploration of problems. The involvement factor is of paramount importance in the discovery process. Involvement is intense. Interruptions are kept at a minimum. Some trial and error is involved in the discovery process. This is part of the learning process. It helps the learner to understand the problem and to begin to delimit the numbers of alternatives which are justifiable for solving the problem. How does discovery differ from other learning activities in its ability to foster creativity? Discovery is more likely to result in the goal of creative behavior because it places the learner and the problem in close proximity while allowing the learner the flexibility and time to explore the situation based on strategies which he/she selects as useful for solving the identified problem. Under these conditions, the learner usually draws on past experiences that helped to solve similar problems as well as intutitive feelings about particular alternatives and their potential for problem resolution. The discovery process is free from the bias of outsiders, therefore, the learner is not hampered by competing ideas of others as he/she grapples with the problem. The intense involvement of the learner draws upon his inner resources and stimulates the mind to make the necessary connections to bring out creative solutions which are rewarding enligtenments for the learner. Satisfaction with the learning process is increased through the discovery process, and creativity is intimately connected with this satisfaction factor.

Clinical Assignments

The student and faculty facilitator plan clinical assignments together in order for the student to feel involved in and enthusiastic about the educational process. In addition, the student is encouraged to plan the nursing care of the client by collaboration with the client and his/her significant others. One of the main components of the creative problem-solving process is the generation of many alternatives. The client is then able to select the alternative(s) which best meet his/her needs, wishes, and goals. The student's learning is enhanced by participation in the process by

FIGURE 11-1
NURSING PROCESS AND CREATIVE PROBLEM SOLVING

Assessing	Planning	Implementing	Evaluation
Fact-finding	Idea-finding Problem-finding	Idea-finding Solution-finding	Acceptance- finding

becoming aware of the alternatives which the client prefers in a given situation. The student learns that it is sometimes necessary to generate additional alternatives before a client is satisfied to select or accept any of the potential alternatives. The need to keep generating new alternatives stretches the mind and frees the student to keep exploring new possibilities. This concept can be illustrated in the following example.

EXAMPLE

Mary Jones is a junior nursing student enrolled in an upper division baccalaureate program. She is taking the second clinical nursing course. She selected a hospitalized white female, age 67 years, with a medical diagnosis of diabetes mellitus as her client. Her health history reveals numerous hospitalizations for insulin and diet regulation, a surgical correction of an ulcer of the foot two years ago, and the usual childhood diseases without complications.

The student is using the nursing process—assessing, planning, implementing, and evaluation—as a basis for nursing interactions. In addition, the creative problem-solving process is used to supplement the nursing process model. It is a five step process: fact-finding, idea-finding, problem-finding, solution-finding, and acceptance-finding. The way the two processes dovetail is illustrated in Figure 11-1

The initial broad statement of the problem the student identified was: How to help Mrs. Jones assume responsibility for the management of her diabetes? In the initial stage of the student-client interaction as many facts as possible related to the situation are gathered. The client's chart is utilized as a valuable adjunct to the interview and physical examination. The facts are listed below:

white female
67 years of age
one cousin living four blocks away
other distant relatives live beyond commuting vicinity

lives alone
efficiency apartment
has two insulin syringes
has six hypodermic needles
speaks and reads English
dislikes cooking
has diabetic diet plans
walks approximately 1/2 mile per week
sits most of day watching TV
bathes once a week
wears sandles and knee length stockings
weighs 120 pounds
height is 5 ft. 3 in.
blood sugar—210 on admission
blood sugar—170 today
insulin 45 U daily
blood pressure 140/80
T-100^8 P-92 R-26 on admission
T-99 P-84 R-24 today
skin dry and flaky
uses eye glasses for reading
dentures
Medicare recipient

The list of facts can be expanded during the other steps of the creative problem-solving process. Each fact is verified with the client.

> *Facts do not cease to exist because they are ignored.*
> Aldous Huxley

The planning phase of the nursing process is promoted by the idea-finding and problem-finding steps of the creative problem-solving process. The *ideas* are generated by brainstorming with the client (and significant others, if appropriate) and by brainstorming with other health professionals responsible for the client's management. At this stage, the quantity of ideas is the major goal rather than the quality of the ideas.

The ideas generated from the brainstorming session between Mrs. Jones and the student included:

1) Make a chart to mark each day when insulin is given
2) Make a meal plan for each day of the week—have three different weekly plans
3) Explore availability of foods that do not need cooking
4) Buy a microwave oven

5) Buy TV dinners
6) Eat at a neighbor's
7) Invite cousin to eat three times a week
8) Plan meals to coincide with TV programs
9) Discourage snacks
10) Have meals on wheels
11) Request vitamins from physician
12) Have ounce of dry wine 1/2 hour before meals
13) Set table with tablecloth and candles
14) Play quiet music at mealtime
15) Explore eating out at Senior Citizen locations, church, hospital dining rooms
16) Prepare week's meals in one day
17) Invite the cousin to prepare the week's meals
18) Advertize for an elderly male to come cook the meals
19) Call the local high school and challenge the cooking class to prepare her meals as a class project
20) Ask the nutritionist to help her plan her meals

The ideas generated from the brainstorming with other health professionals included the following additional ideas (ideas which were the same as in the other list are omitted from this list).

1) Have her prepare her meals while in the hospital
2) Have her eat her meals in the hospital cafeteria
3) Have her cousin come to share meals with her in hospital
4) Contact minister at local church to come visit
5) Have minister identify potential visitors from congregation
6) Have visiting nurse visit three times a week
7) Home health aide daily for four hours
8) Advertise for adolescent to come for meals
9) Identify a person to call her each day at mealtimes

The health team wanted some additional facts so the student asked Mrs. Jones the questions to obtain these additional facts.

periodically attends church
Baptist
church within four blocks of home
enjoys church
does not have any special friends at church
does not know the minister very well
minister has not visited her home
minister does not know she has diabetes and is hospitalized frequently

does not know if there are any church groups which interest her
would like the student to instigate communication with the minister

The planning phase is also promoted by the second step of the creative problem solving; the statement of the problem is expressed in a creative format. In this stage, the client is asked to review the list of ideas and identify the ones that are most attractive to her. The ideas identified by Mrs. Jones as most attractive are listed below:

buy a microwave oven
explore eating out
contact minister

The statement of these ideas in problem-solving format results in the following statements for Mrs. Jones:

How might I buy a microwave oven?
How might I contact the minister to help?
How might I eat out?

The student shares the restatement of the problem with Mrs. Jones. Mrs. Jones verifies that the questions are ones she would like to work on.

The creative problem-solving process continues by brainstorming ways to find solutions to the three questions with the help of Mrs. Jones. This brainstorming is part of the planning stage in the nursing process model. The goal in this brainstorming session is to generate as many ideas as possible. Judgment is still deferred. The brainstorming session produced the following.

Regarding the microwave:

1) Take up a collection
2) Use savings
3) Buy chances on a raffle
4) Share expenses with cousin
*5) Shop for best buy
*6) Watch the ads for sales
*7) Watch the ads for second hand one
8) Make one
9) Use the one at hospital snack bar
10) Join a club that has one
11) Send a request to Santa Claus
12) Wish for one
13) Steal one
14) Rent one
15) Buy an oven toaster
16) Move to an apartment that has one
17) Share one with a neighbor

*18) Give $12.00 a month towards the purchase

*19) Charge one

The alternatives chosen by Mrs. Jones (identified by *) as most likely to be possible are numbers 5, 6, 7, 18, and 19. (Note, judgment is made after the brainstorming session is completed.)

The student and Mrs. Jones then brainstormed ideas in relation to the second question. The list of ideas from the question related to the minister follow:

  1) Have Mrs. Jones call him

*2) Have the student call him

  3) Have the cousin stop by to see him

  4) Send him a note

  5) Leave a message for him with the telephone operator

  6) Visit the church after discharge

*7) Get a pass to visit the minister

*8) Have the student go with Mrs. Jones to the minister

  9) Have the student visit the minister

10) Watch for him in the hospital and stop him

11) Contact a member of the church and have her talk to him

12) Wait unitl discharge and give Mrs. Jones his telephone number

13) Have Mrs. Jones stop by the church on her way home from the hospital

14) Have social service call him

15) Send a courier pigeon

16) Whistle

17) Have a party and invite him over

18) Have him bring a microwave oven

19) Advertize in the paper

20) Send a donation

The alternatives chosen by Mrs. Jones as most likely to hold the most promise are numbers 2, 7, and 8.

Next, the brainstorming session centered on the third question. Mrs. Jones wanted ideas on how she could eat out. The ideas follow:

  1) Get a boyfriend to pay

*2) Find inexpensive restaurants

  3) Establish a meal plan at a local restaurant

  4) Seek a discount for weekly meals

*5) Use hospital cafeteria

  6) Go with cousin

  7) Brown bag it in the park

  8) Brown bag it anywhere you like

9) Purchase it from mobile meal truck
10) Eat out twice a week
11) Eat dinner at home, other meals out
12) Eat dinner out, other meals at home
13) Visit a neighbor at meal time
14) Volunteer in high school cafeteria in exchange for lunch
*15) Volunteer in hospital snack bar in exchange for lunch
16) Select new interesting restaurant to visit each week
17) Join a restaurant club
18) Join a country club
19) Bring brown bag and purchase things you like but would not cook yourself
20) Save $5 from each check to treat yourself
21) Organize a progressive meal with friends
22) Start a club for sharing meals in each other's homes
23) Take a lottery ticket each month

The ideas that Mrs. Jones selected as most feasible are numbers 2, 5, and 15.

During the implementation phase of the nursing process, the student generates ideas to facilitate the options Mrs. Jones selected for achieving her goals. Mrs. Jones and the student plan together so the implementation progresses smoothly. Mrs. Jones is asked to decide which questions have the highest priority for her. She decided that her highest priority was to involve the minister. Her next selection was the purchase of the microwave and the third was how to eat out. Therefore the list of ideas, based on priority, is now:

Have the student call the minister
Get a pass to visit the minister
Have the student go with Mrs. Jones to visit the minister
Shop for best buy on a microwave
Watch the ads for sales on microwaves
Watch the ads for second hand microwaves
Save $12.00 a month towards the purchase of a microwave
Charge the microwave
Find inexpensive restaurants
Use the hospital cafeteria
Volunteer in hospital snack bar in exchange for lunch

The following plan for implementation was established:

The student telephones the minister for an appointment immediately. Mrs. Jones asks the physician for a pass to visit the minister on the appointed day. The student talks to her/his instructor about the plan.

The purchase of the microwave warranted further deliberation. The ideas, selected by Mrs. Jones, did not give a clear explanation of her wishes. Some of the ideas would result in purchasing the microwave now while others indicated a desire to delay the purchase. The student and Mrs. Jones discussed the situation further. Mrs. Jones decided that she could not buy the microwave on a delayed payment plan. Instead, Mrs. Jones decided to keep watch of advertisements and to save the money for a later purchase.

Next, the student and Mrs. Jones decided on a plan to implement the goal of eating out. The student contacted the director of the volunteer services. She talked with Mrs. Jones about her desire to be a volunteer in exchange for receiving free lunch. The director was delighted and planned for Mrs. Jones to be a volunteer on Mondays and Fridays. Mrs. Jones decided that she would eat dinner at the hospital cafeteria at her own expense on Tuesday, Thursdays, and Saturdays. The hospital dietitian was contacted. She was given a copy of Mrs. Jones' schedule. She discussed Mrs. Jones food preferences with her. Then she devised a diet plan to facilitate Mrs. Jones' plan. Next, the student and Mrs. Jones made a list of all the restaurants in the neighborhood. Some of the restaurants were listed in a community restaurant guide. It was easy to cross off the restaurants which Mrs. Jones could not afford to use as they had expensive ratings in the listing. The remaining restaurants Mrs. Jones was asked to rate based on her assessment. She was familiar with some of them while others were unfamiliar. She planned to call the unfamiliar restaurants when she returned home to finalize the list of restaurants she would use when she did not feel like cooking.

The next phase in the nursing process is *evaluation*. The corresponding stage in the creative problem-solving stage is *acceptance-finding*. At this time, it is important to establish a realistic timetable for completing the plan. It is also necessary to judge the outcomes of actions that have been completed. In this instance, the evaluation is delayed to see if the action results in better regulation of Mrs. Jones' diabetic condition. The only thing that can be evaluated at this time are some of the *means* established to meet the *end* goal. The actions taken to make contact with the minister and the volunteer director are positive steps for helping to alleviate the problems. However, unless the follow-up is productive, Mrs. Jones' diabetic condition would remain unaltered by the action. Therefore, the student planned a telephone follow-up call to Mrs. Jones. She planned to have lunch with Mrs. Jones on the first day that Mrs. Jones worked as a volunteer. She also planned to join Mrs. Jones for dinner in the hospital cafeteria on the following Thursday. The student arranged to be present for Mrs. Jones' follow-up clinic visit scheduled three weeks after her discharge. At the clinic visit, the student could gather data about Mrs. Jones' physical condition and talk with her about the plan they established.

DISCUSSION

The client-student interaction is strengthened by the process of brainstorming. Through this process, the client feels actively involved in the planning of care. The process allows the client to choose the alternatives that are most attractive and then the student and client, together, decide on a plan for implementation. The client maintains a great deal of control in this process. The student acts as a facilitator and readily withdraws when the client is ready to assume full responsibility for the selected course of action. The student does not assume total responsibility for deciding what is best for the client in contrast to how client-care is often planned. Furthermore, the creative problem-solving process allows for a broader look at problems and their potential resolution.

Mrs. Jones' initial problem of noncompliance with the diabetic regime seems less threatening when it is approached in a creative way. The student benefits personally by knowing he/she is fostering independence in clients and benefits professionally by being privileged to help a client resolve a health problem. The process also demonstrates to the student that there are many alternatives that are acceptable for solving problems. As all the alternativies emerge, the client has more possibilities available to select from. The student has the advantage of being a first hand witness to the alternatives selected by clients when they are presented with opportunities to choose their own course of action for resolving their health problems.

A student involved in this process is freed from the need to memorize a list of potential solutions to problems. The student is allowed the freedom to take each problem that arises and have it solved by a specific plan geared to the individual client.

The student views each experience with a client as a challenge to be explored to its fullest, seeing each client as a fascinating and unique individual with a whole compilation of experiences that make the client an outstanding creation. As a creation, a work of art, the client has beauties, has faults, has potential for change, has the ability to arouse feelings in others, and has qualities that set him/her apart from other similar works of art.

The wonderment that surrounds each client acts as a stimulus to the student to want to get inside the client, to fully understand him/her as a person rather than the person the student wishes him to be. The students learn to relate to each person as he/she really is. Clients are often viewed from what others wish they were, and this posture interferes with the full understanding of persons as they are. When a client and student come together, the student has a supreme opportunity to feel, at the gut level, the true person, the person who is before him/her, the person who can unfold experiences that make him what what he is today. The unfolding process helps the student to understand why the outer cover is encased in hostility or frustration, beauty or contentment, or suspicion and rejection. The student has the privilege of being able to learn from the client while delivering nursing services as part of the health care sought by the client. Too often the delivery of services interferes with obtaining the full essence of who the client is and robs both the student and client of opportunities to share in living life more fully. The least valued human being in society is not without experiences that would help us understand *human functioning* which is the heart and lungs of our chosen profession. Therefore, the study of the human being is the primary goal of each student experience. The student is held accountable for understanding the client as the client unfolds and projects himself/herself. Inferences about the client are kept to a minimum. The joy felt by drawing premature inferences must be replaced by a joy that is associated with really knowing the client from the client's point of view. An illustration follows:

> A client comes to the gynecological clinic on pregnancy termination day in a cotton print, loosely flowing dress with torn tennis shoes, oily, stringy brown hair, dull eyes, somber face, and the smell of perspiration penetrating from her body.
>
> The physician reviews the client's old records and notes that she had two previous elective abortions. Her current record indicates that she is four weeks pregnant and desires another abortion. The physician is angered by the record and the woman's appearance and decides that she will not get an abortion through his clinic.
>
> The student most likely will not be able to change the physician's decision. However, there are opportunities for the student to listen to the client unfold her story. The outer cover, which angered the physician, is not allowed to interfere with the student/client interaction. It is only through describing, without judging, that the clients and their choices can be fully understood. The biases which prevail within professional groups cannot be used to determine what students will learn about each unique individual. Listening to the client will help the student see the relationship between the client who is sitting beside him/her and the client the physician, and perhaps the student, wishes she was. The discrepancy between these two images needs to be dealt with in a constructive way if students are to learn to appreciate the client as a creative work of art.

Conclusion

The nursing profession is dependent on today and tomorrow's students to guarantee its continued existence. Students, helped to use creative potential, will develop skills in problem-solving that will help them become effective and competent nursing practitioners. The educational experiences offered to students is based on a process orientation which helps students toward a broader understanding of the field and provides opportunities for students to be intimately involved in the educational process.

The educational process needs to provide opportunities for students to become sensitive and selective in their use of the imagination and its relationship to the world of fact and reality.[2]

Chapter 12

Nurturing
Creative Potential of Clients

The example of the student-client interaction can also be used to illustrate how the creative potential of clients is fostered by the creative problem-solving process.

The nurse is not able to fully understand the *real self* of clients. However, by demonstrating a willingness to become part of the client's world, by providing support and strength, the nurse participates in the client's ability to assume self-growth. The *real self* of individuals is extremely complex, defying simple intrusions into it; therefore, the nurse interacts with a client, temporarily trying to understand the private and inner feelings which influence the way he/she responds to the health or illness state. In order for the client to continue to grow, he/she needs to maintain the uniqueness of self and receive positive reinforcement for that self. It becomes imperative that the interventions planned with or on behalf of the client seek to maintain rather than destroy the uniqueness of self.

As Moustakas[1] clearly identifies, only the individual person has the ability to actualize his/her own potential. To accomplish this goal, it is necessary to learn and to grow. This learning and growing leads to self-identity. The ability to grow is influenced by physical as well as emotional factors. Intrinsic biological factors influence the individual's ability to function effectively. Or as Moustakas suggests, the nurturing and cultivation of the intrinsic factors affect one's ability to maintain personal integrity which leads towards expression of individuality and self-actualization. Members of the nursing profession have the expertise to foster the cultivation and nurturance of both the intrinsic and extrinsic factors related to self-actualization of the clients who select or are referred to their services.

The strategy of nurses is to focus on the "who-ness" rather than the "what-ness" of clients, or stated another way, the focus is on who the client is and not on what he/she is. There must be a definite attempt by professionals not to force their personal and professional convictions and values on the client lest we impair the client's ability for creativity and therefore limit his/her will to explore and to self-actualize.

The total emersion of one's self in another person's situation without losing one's own identity allows each participant to experience a sense of oneness, a singleness of purpose which makes the coming together a rewarding experience. The close encounter between client and provider sets the stage for the client to feel the freedom to explore new horizons, breaking away from the behaviors that prohibit the exploration of using new alternatives for resolving life's problems.

Maintaining Identity

The client's right to express his/her own identity is essential to the client being himself/herself. The professionals, responsible for guiding care, have an obligation to be certain that clients are free to express their unique identity. In order to insure the client the freedom to express identity, the environment needs to be free of punitive attitudes of health care professionals. The expression of identity is very important to the child who is still learning who he/she is in relation to the world. The child health nurse facilitates the expression of identity by limiting authoritarian postures, by keeping orders at a minimum, and by helping the child to select and control the things he/she wants to do. The child who is hospitalized needs to be given choices to help him/her feel that the plan of care will result in self-integrity as well as a return to a healthy state of being. Clients of all ages are given the opportunity to grow in human relations when the rules and regulations are kept at a minimum and individualization of care is focused on the client as a unique individual. The interaction between clients and professionals must include a respect for one another and a realization that conformity to demands and expectations result in alienation rather than in cooperation. As Moustakas[2] wisely notes, self-denial and self-neglect lead to maladaptive rather than adaptive behavior. Self-denial and self-neglect tend to destroy the self of the client. The client needs to feel important in the professionals' world, not an afterthought or a roadblock. The environments where health care is administered need to be restructured until the goal of client-centered care and total client care become a reality. In client-centered facilities it is easier for clients to maintain and express their identity.

Zinker[3] points out that it is necessary to have a variety of experiences in order for creativity to flourish. The client who lacks opportunities to experience life in an expanded fashion may be less capable of creative expression, if this is the case. While nursing cannot promise each client the probability of enriching life experiences through art, music, dance, and so forth, we can deepen the client's experiences by becoming involved in human interactions with our clients through displaying a sincere interest in their problems and building a bond of trust between the client, nurse, and the health care system. Nursing cannot assume total responsibility for all clients not being born equal, but we can assume an obligation to treat each person as equal when we deliver nursing services.

Occasionally it is also important to inspire people, to model the full range of humaneness which jolts them into goals they never understood, much less considered.[3]

Creative Problem Solving

The client can be intimately involved in the creative problem-solving process. Involvement in the problem-solving process negates the client being placed in a passive position and care being planned without his/her involvement. Involving the client in care planning is a way to increase awareness and prove that his/her contributions are vital to the successful implementation of the health plan. The client is held accountable for choosing alternatives that are reasonable and attainable but is not held accountable for always selecting the best alternative. Brainstorming ideas as part of problem-solving sessions usually produce ideas that the client would not consider under the ordinary circumstances which surround the delivery of health care. When faced with the need to generate ideas, the client, as well as professionals, think of things that are not traditionally chosen. The process of brainstorming purges the mind. This purging helps to generate creative ideas. In addition to the brainstorming strategy, purging can also be accomplished in this way: (Note, inflections in the nurse's voice are by italics.)

EXAMPLE

The client says that he has a problem taking his medications on time.
Professional: Why is this a problem?
    Client: Because I don't feel good when I forget the medication.
Professional: *Why* is this a problem?
    Client: Because I need the medication to live.
Professional: Why is *that* a problem?
    Client: Because my family can't survive without me.
Professional: *Why* is that a problem?
    Client: Because my wife doesn't work.
Professional: *How* is that a problem?
    Client: She is dependent on me.
Professional: Is that a *problem?*
    Client: Yes, it makes me very uncomfortable.
Professional: *How* does it make you uncomfortable?
    Client: I feel jittery all the time.

Professional: How is *that* a problem?
     Client: It puts added stress on me.
Professional: *How* is that a problem?
     Client: I forget things when I'm upset.
Professional: *How* is that a problem?
     Client: I feel frustrated whan I forget things.
Professional: Do you forget your medication more often when you are
           under this stress?
     Client: Yes

DISCUSSION

After this purging session, it is easier to establish a plan for the client to take medications. The client is now aware that part of the problem is due to stress levels and a plan to resolve or decrease stress must be incorporated into the plan of action. Frequently clients are not fully aware of the associations between their current problem and other things. The creative problem-solving process attempts to help them explore the situation from a broader base.

Clients also need to be encouraged to see that the solution to their problems frequently lies within their own resources. It is the role of the health professional to provide encouragement and reinforcement so the client feels comfortable and capable to find the solutions to his/her own problems.

Providing the client with sufficient opportunity to explore the pathways available to him/her before giving solutions based on past "truths" and professional bias is providing the client with the freedom to test his/her own hypotheses before generating inferences about what will or will not happen. The supportive nature of the provider helps the client continue to benefit from the *process* of problem solving. The eventual creation of a solution is an exhilarating experience arising from the inner resources of the client rather than being superimposed by someone else. Or as Zinker[3] suggests, creating change in one's life is taking the risk to release one's self, one's heart and soul, into the world. The freedom to express the fantasies, desires, and thoughts which invade our minds is part of the exhilarating experience of living life to its fullest in spite of the criticism or rejection that it might cause.

Creativity of Clients

Creativity can be generated by having the client's environment changed. The use of music is an effective stimulus for some clients. The problem-solving session is interrupted briefly and music is introduced. The music can be of any variety. It does not have to be music that the client generally prefers in order to be effective. Five or ten minutes of rock, western, contemporary, classical, etc, can be just the interlude that helps to stimulate additional creative thought. In conjunction with the music, the client can smell cotton pligits moistened with sweet, pungent, familiar, and unfamiliar smells. There is no magic way to predict which music or scents might result in creative thought, so variability is suggested. Clients can assume the responsibility for introducing music (auditory stimulus) and odors (olfactory stimulus) themselves whenever they feel that their thought processes are slowing down. The clinic, office, and hospital settings where clients and professionals engage in planning for health management are rarely conducive to quiet thinking which can be valuable in stimulating creative thought. A walk outside to see the grass, sky, or flowers is helpful to counteract the sterile settings. The client is encouraged to pay special attention to nature by concentrating on the beauty and mystical qualities of nature. Some clients value this type of experience while others do not value it. It is essential to explain the rationale for the suggestion and then let the client decide whether to do it. It must be emphasized that persons who do not value the activity are probably not able to reap benefits from participating in this way.

Another way to nurture creative behavior in the client population is through the use of films. The long waiting times in clinics can be used to show a combination of health films and creative films. (A list of creative films appears in Appendix A.)

Many activities that encourage creative action are fun. This is why clients are usually receptive to trying them. The vestibular and tactile senses can be sharpened by use of exercises put to music. A charming record with directions for participation is "Get Fit While You Sit." A list of records appears in Appendix B. A more vigorous activity is parachute play. A parachute (or similar round nylon piece of material) is used in combination with music to encourage movement. A note of caution is essential here. It is best to have the physician's approval for clients with respiratory, cardiac, or movement problems to participate in this activity. Clients can participate from wheelchairs as well as from a standing position. The parachute play encourages group participation and comraderie. The vigorous parachute play can be followed by a period of relaxation fostered by relaxation techniques. Clients able to lie on the floor are encouraged to begin by relaxing their toes and then proceeding to relax each body part progressing upwards towards and including the head. A few minutes of relaxed comfort and then the leader begins the instructions to wake up the body parts beginning at the head and reversing the process ending with the toes. The increasing emphasis placed on exercise and its relationship to physical fitness and healthy living makes this type of activity seem very appropriate in a health care facility. It is fortunate that exercise, relaxation, and meditation are all connected with nurturing creative potential.

Many clients, but most certainly children, are likely to benefit by creating stories. There are at least two ways to stimulate this creative process. One way is to list many nouns and then to direct the client to write a story using all the listed words and any other he/she wishes to include. The words act as a stimulus to the person to produce the story.

EXERCISES

EXERCISE 1

The following list of words is placed on a chalkboard, flannelboard, 8½ x 11 sheet of white paper, or on the back of an old envelope.

dog	door	plant	airplane
cat	wheelbarrow	witch	roof
bicycle	chair	robber	door
cart	furnace	water	oven
tree	basket	orange cat	policeman
refrigerator	table	pot	escalator
milkman	fireman	pan	librarian
baby	old man	fairy godmother	fence

If there is a group of clients who are participating, each one is asked to use the list of words in a different way. The first person is assigned the first column. He/she is directed to use the words as they appear, starting at the top and working down through the word *baby*. The next person can be directed to start at the bottom and work up. Each column can be assigned in this way. If there are more persons other combinations can be suggested such as using the first two words in each column, or using the last two words, or letting them use any eight words they choose, or using every other word, etc. The key issue is to have the client have the benefit of words which help to stimulate him/her to produce a story. Without the stimulus words, persons sometimes feel like they are unable to produce a story.

The second way to help create stories follows.

EXERCISE 2:

Five columns are drawn and headed by the words: HERO, HEROINE, VILLAIN, TIME, PLACE. Then, the group is asked to brainstorm ten things to put in each column. For example:

146

	HERO	HEROINE	VILLAIN	TIME	PLACE
1)	Uncle Sam	Betty Freidan	Big Bad Wolf	1880	Outer space
2)	Tarzan	Flo Nightengale	Cookie Monster	2 AM	On mountain top
3)	Batman	Roselyn Carter	Frankenstein	6 PM	In the water
4)	Kojak	Farrah Fawcett	Tax Collector	Today	In jail
5)	President Carter	Bionic Woman	Bandit	1744	haunted house
6)	Begin	Minny Mouse	Thief	Future	In this room
7)	Dr. DeBakey	Madam Curie	Car Thief	1979	In the hospital
8)	McArthur	Alice in Wonderland	Hijacker	Midnight	In a mansion
9)	Joe Namath	Barbara Jordan	Wicked step-mother	Morning	Alaska
10)	O.J. Simpson	Cinderella	Dracula	Late	In a school

It is necessary to select one word from each column. This can be done by asking someone to give their telephone number without the area code. As the number is given, the leader encircles the appropriate item. For instance, the number 488-2643 is given. The story will revolve around:

4. Kojack—Hero
8. Alice in Wonderland—Heroine
8. Hijacker—Villain
2. 2 AM—Time
6. In this room—Place

Each person writes a story using the same words. The stories can be shared and if time permits, they can be acted out as well. Another variation of this activity is to select a producer and have that person design the story and cast participants as actors or as props in the story. Another variation of this exercise is to have each person use his/her own telephone number to select the words and write a story. This results in a wider variety of stories to share with the group or to act out.

DISCUSSION

Activities of this type help to make the time spent in hospitals or waiting rooms more tolerable. Some of the activities are more suited to particular clients than to others. The main thing to keep in mind is that being creative involves a change in perspective. Exercises like the ones provided help to convince people that they possess creative thought. The creative professional is eager is provide opportunities for creativity to emerge in clients.

Self-Help

The client is more aware that it is possible to assume increased responsibility for maintaining and restoring his/her own health. The client is aided in self-help activity by the use of books specifically written for this purpose and by health professionals committed to the concept of self-help.

It takes a certain amount of creativity to assume the self-help role in relation to one's health. Areas related to health that lend themselves to self-help techniques are nutrition, exercise, birth, minor illnesses, and so forth. The clients that are successful in self-help activities are likely to be eager to use creativity in their self-help endeavors. The nursing profession has an unending responsibility to encourage and support clients in their self-help activities. The means used by clients to achieve self-help methodologies need to be explored by professionals. A great deal of value can be learned from these clients and their creative approaches to health maintenance and restoration. Two examples help to illustrate this point. A client with a painful low back strain suspended ropes from his cellar rafters and exercised to increase the strength in his back muscles. The pain from the back strain disappeared. The exercise program was designed through trail and error using his own resources and was very effective. Creative ideas like the one described can be shared with other clients who have similar health problems and desire a self-help approach. In this situation, the client had the permission of his physician to try the exercises. A physical examination is indicated before another client would be encouraged to try the self-help plan to be certain that a serious health problem is not causing the back pain.

Recently, an inventor described his creative product for treating tennis elbow. An avid tennis player, his painful elbow interfered with his game. He tried several traditional remedies for the condition without success. Then, by trial and error, he devised a product that was successful in relieving the tension. He experimented with a variety of materials and finally achieved his goal. The creative product is useful and is selling to many other tennis hopefuls who have the same painful affliction.

Just as the examples in the student-client interactions relate to nurturing creative potential in both groups, the examples in the client section are equally valuable for encouraging creativity in students.

Chapter 13

Nurturing Creativity in Nurse Managers

The job of the nurse manager requires a sense of perspective and flexibility of thought and action. The positions are often filled with generous amounts of frustrations and disappointments. In order to maintain a sense of achievement, managers need a way to infiltrate the system and to generate positive experiences for themselves and for their employees. A creative person is likely to achieve the goal of being a successful nurse manager.

Ackoff[1] identifies the five C's of the properties associated with good management: *competence, communicativeness, concern, courage,* and *creativity.* He suggests that creativity is the greatest of the group. He proposes that without creativity the organization can be managed effectively, but it cannot move ahead of other organizations, it merely remains as one organization among many. He proposes that managers are poorly prepared for their positions because teachers tend not to teach creativity and courage. (See also page 50.) Managers who lack these two attributes are in a disadvantaged position to manage effectively.

A problem frequently evades a solution because incorrect assumptions are made that preclude successful resolution.[1] We tend to solve problems as though there was only one potential solution to each problem. This approach results in a person searching for the answers proposed by another rather than looking for alternatives that might result in creative solutions. To allow creativity to emerge, we need to be freed from the assumptions that place constraints on problem solving.

Ackoff[1] defines the difference between *reactive* and *proactive* problem solving. Reactive problem solving is a retrospective process, while proactive problem solving is aimed at getting something that is wanted. The majority of problem solving falls into the category of retroactive problem solving, while a more productive situation is to engage in proactive problem solving.

The roles of nurse managers are extremely diverse. However, in almost every role, the nurse manager interacts with a large number of persons with divergent personalities. The nurse manager attempts to fertilize the soil so that associates can grow in their positions. In a sense, the role is similar to the role of the nurse faculty-facilitator. The greatest difference between the role of the nurse manager and the nurse faculty-facilitator is that the people the nurse manager attempts to help grow usually include a wider range of educational preparation, life experiences, personal goals, and so forth, than the persons that faculty facilitators are involved with. It is not unusual for the nurse manager to coordinate the outputs of volunteers, aides, paraprofessionals, and other nurses with varying qualifications and a variety of other health care workers. The role is to *manage* and to make the system work effectively. No small charge!

> How can two equally competent people look at the same situation with the same data, one see only problems or just a routine assignment, the other see a whole cluster of open-ended new profit possibilities? How can two equally intelligent, motivated and well-informed managers come upon the same problem—and one be stuck with that problem for long, costly years, the other immediately see and apply creative solutions which open up new opportunities for advance? The difference is: creativity and initiative!

It is easy to hypothesize that the nurse manager will be aided in endeavors if he/she possesses the attributes of a creative person. MacKinnon[3] summarizes that these persons have an unusual capacity to record, retain, and recall life experiences. In addition, they observe situations in a different way. They are alert to challenges and tend to be able to shift their attention easily from one situation to a new situation. They are able to draw upon their thoughts and bring forth those that serve to solve the problems they face. These attributes, combined with the large repertoire of knowledge, facilitate their involvement in problem-solving situations. Based on these characteristics, it seems evident that nurse managers should be helped to develop their creative potential in order to increase their ability and skills in relation to *identifying* problem situations and helping to solve the problems in a creative way.

The ability to sense problems before they become crisis situations is an art. The creative person explores the environment to identify problems or challenges rather than attempting to ignore these situations hoping they will go away. The creative manager, therefore, does not spend the majority of the time going around putting out fires. Instead, the kindling timbers are viewed as challenges before the fire is started. This situation allows the nurse manager time to involve the staff in creative problem-solving methodologies, while a crisis format situation does not use this approach. Or to use MacKinnon's[3] words, the creative person is intuitively alert to the possibilities that may occur and to things which are not yet realized. This facility puts the creative person in a good position to accept the responsibilities of managing systems.

If the hypothesis that creative persons will be more effective managers is believed, then nurse managers should not be chosen through a process consistent with the Peter Principle.* Instead they should be selected on the basis of their life experiences, body of knowledge, and creative tendencies. The ongoing education of nurse-managers should reflect an emphasis on nurturing their creative potential rather than on instructional programs which focus on how to structure the environment in order to gain and keep control. A rigid controlled environment is not conducive to the development of creative employees.

Meetings

How, then, is it possible for the nurse manager to maintain a semblance of order, be ready to bring calm out of chaos, and motivate persons to achieve at a consistently high level of performance? Using a combination of the routine solutions, interspersed with periods of free-flowing ideation, will help to achieve this goal. Specific meeting times for idea generation need to be included in the work schedule or else only the routine aspects of the job will receive attention. Periodically, these meetings can be held away from the institution to provide a neutral environment for rejuvenation to take place. An attempt is made to have these meetings viewed as a positive valuable opportunity to enrich the work experience and to enrich the personal lives of the employees. Otherwise, the meetings may be viewed negatively, and this affective response interferes with the effectiveness of the meeting.

If MacKinnon's[3] work is accepted, creative persons value truth and esthetics. While this combination sometimes produces conflicts, the creative person has the adaptability to successfully resolve the conflict. Truth and esthetics are both included in the meeting environment. Many of the activities suggested in the other sections of this book are used to provide the esthetic component of the program. In addition, the workshop atmosphere is planned to provide positive, friendly interactions. An attempt is made to invite the employees to the meeting in novel new ways. The novelty tends to stimulate their interest.

EXAMPLE

A series of invitations are sent; the first one is incomplete, only announcing the date (ie, Save November 25th. More later); the second one is sent a couple of weeks later announcing the place (ie, The Old Mill—November 25!); the third one is sent out a couple weeks before the event (ie:

*Peter LJ, Hull R: The Peter Principle. New York, William Morrow & Co, 1969. A person is promoted until a level of incompetence is reached.

It's almost here!
The Old Mill
November 25, 1978 @ 9 am
The Mind Expander!
You'all come!).

Prior to the assemblege, a theme for the meeting is selected and implemented. A western theme can be executed by having cowboy hats with name tags or name tags shaped like cowboy boots. The lunch can be a western barbeque complete with western music and dancing. Periodic breaks in the "truth" sessions can carry the theme further, such as providing for a game of horseshoes, yodeling contest, and so forth. The decorations in the rooms also reflect the chosen theme. There needs to be a balance of time in the schedule to guarantee that opportunities are provided for using the right and left hemispheres of the brain. Therefore, a tentative schedule of events is provided. The agenda is kept flexible to attempt to meet the individual desires of the participants. The format of the meeting combines individual, dyadic encounters, small group and large group activities as well as periods for meditation, relaxation, and music. The work sessions are related to problems identified by employees and ones identified by the nurse manager.

DISCUSSION

The meetings are intended to be enjoyable and productive. If the meeting is successful, employees and managers both express satisfaction with being a part of the interaction and are motivated to implement the ideas which are generated. Between meetings the manager builds in connections with the experience to help the employees see the relationship of what they are doing in the day to day work situation with what they experienced in the meetings. If the connections are not established, some of the vitality gained through the experience is lost. The greatest value gained from the workshop format meeting is that the hours spent during the workshop result in viable solutions for problems in the work situation.

The workshop format, away from the troubling aspects of the job, is a better environment for encouraging creative thinking. The literal break from the agency seems to hasten the break from the traditional ways of thinking and problem solving. In addition, the barriers which build up between employees and managers can be overcome easier outside the structure of the agency. Also, it is more acceptable to combine work with pleasure in a neutral setting.

It is not possible for all employees or managers to feel comfortable in the nontraditional meeting. Therefore, it is wise to spend time explaining the rationale for the meeting with these people. They may never come to accept the idea, but they may learn to tolerate it more easily.

Role Modeling

The nurse manager acts as a role model for establishing positive morale in associates. High morale is achieved by keeping a proper balance between satisfaction with the current situation and at the same time possessing a posture of constructive discontent with the setting. When the nurse manager detects dissatisfaction, possible alternatives for improving the situation are proposed. The successful nurse manager is not content to identify negative situations and habitually complain about them. Instead, he/she tries to look at the situation in a more positive framework. The positive attitude should not take on a "Pollyanna" aura, however. The nurse manager who is too positive in a situation infiltrated with many problems loses credibility with colleagues. Positive attitudes, when viewed by others as sincere, are infectious. It is exciting to have positive rather than negative attitudes spread through the organization.

The role model behaviors of the nurse manager extend beyond fostering high morale in colleagues. Role modeling requires competence in dealing with disputes, demonstrating skill in delivering nursing services, effectively collaborating with other health care providers, and being knowledgeable about clinical practice as well as management techniques. In order to fill these demands, the nurse-manager must be qualified academically, professionally, and personally. Knowledge without personal or professional credibility will not adequately prepare the nurse manager to function as a role model. Likewise, professional and personal qualifications without academic qualifications leaves the nurse manager in a disadvantaged position for assuming the role.

Patient Care Conferences

A vital part of nursing care relates to client care conferences. The nurse manager facilitates this activity on the client units. The goal of these conferences is to improve the quality of nursing care. The conferences are usually structured around clients with special problems and necessitate a thorough exploration of the situation. The nurse manager helps the staff improve their skills in relation to the creative resolution of problems. In addition to using the five step creative problem-solving method identified in Chapter 7, the nurse manager uses methodologies for improving group process. The methodologies in Chapter 6 are appropriate and an additional example follows.

EXAMPLE

The use of the fish bowl technique for focusing on participants' contributions to the group is suggested. An inner and outer circle are established. The persons in the inner circle are assigned a problem to discuss. The persons in the outer circle are assigned one person in the inner circle on which to focus. Thus, each person in the inner circle has an outside observer. The role of the observer is to note the verbal and nonverbal contributions of a specific observee in the group. When the discussion is completed, the observer and observee come together and discuss what took place. After this discussion, they return to the circle. This time the person in the inner circle tries to improve the contributions to the discussion based on the feedback from the observer. After this session they again discuss as a dyad the changes in group participation behavior. Then they change roles and complete the same process.

DISCUSSION

The role of team members in client care conferences are strengthened by this procedure. If attempts are not made to strengthen team conferences, some group members may tend to monopolize the discussion while other members do not contribute a thing. Either of these extremes in behavior tend to decrease the efficiency of the group process. Strengthening group participation skills through the fish bowl technique is a way to get maximum input into the client care conference by making each group member feel that contributions by all members are valued.

Problem Solving and Decision Making

The area of decision-making poses some unique problems for the creative nurse manager. This is due to the criteria used to determine decisions selected by creative persons. According to DiCyan,[4] criteria selected by creative persons for decision making include hunches, individual ideas, innovation, deviation from standard format, speculation, intuition, and feelings. Contrast these criteria with the criteria frequently used in decision-making: surveys and data, team and consensus, precedent, and standards and patterns. It becomes apparent that the creative nurse manager will have some difficulty maintaining credibility if the organization is too traditional. The creative person tends to be thwarted by the bureaucratic red tape which structures conventional decision-making strategies.

The nurse manager role demands skill in problem solving and decision making. This demanding role places the nurse manager in the position of needing many strategies to resolve problems in the work environment. The goal of problem solving and decision making is to consider all the choices that are possible rather than jumping at decisions based on the first idea that comes to mind.

In many situations, there are infinite numbers of alternatives available for consideration. The more complex the situation, the more likely the alternatives will lend themselves to categorization. However, it is necessary to use discretion when forming categories to be certain that good ideas are not lost in the process.

Stevens[5] stresses that nurse managers follow three basic principles to assure that a premature classification of a problem does not occur:

1) know all the relevant data before diagnosing a problem;
2) recognize that most problems relate to interpretation of the facts;
3) systematically investigate the scope of each identified problem.

The nurse manager is alert not to fall into the trap of resolving problems before they are adequately identified. If this happens, the solution results in temporary stability in the situation but the real problem still needs resolution. Therefore, the symptoms of the problem will continue to persist until the real problem is resolved. Stevens[5] offers a model for assessing alternatives for problem solutions. It is a three-sided model focusing on *goals*, *structure*, and *technology*. She proposes that the nurse manager assess the proposed alternative for one part of the model and determine its compatibility with the other two parts of the model. An example, based on this model follows.

EXAMPLE

Goal—The nurse manager on the pediatric in-patient area desires that all new personnel in the pediatric area view the film "Play in the Hospital" before being employed.

Structure—The nurse manager in the pediatric in-patient area does not interview new applicants. They are interviewed by the personnel department and the director of nurses.

Technology—The film is available in the in-service department and the in-service staff are willing to show the film.

DISCUSSION

In this example, the goal and technology are congruent but the structure interferes with the successful achievement of the goal. In order to remedy this situation, the nurse-manager focuses attention on the structure that is negatively controlling the activity. As an example, one alternative is to have the nurse manager also interview new applicants.

Decision Making Regarding Absenteeism

Many of the challenges faced by nurse-managers are considered trivia to an outsider. However, to the individuals intimately involved with the situation, they are extremely important. When challenges seem minor, it is easy to accept solutions without giving the situation reasonable scrutiny. The nurse-manager who chooses this modus operandi is not atypical of other managers, but is still not doing justice to the role. For example, a nurse's aide habitually calls in sick on the Friday prior to her scheduled weekend off duty. The nurse-manager, instead of generating all the alternatives for dealing with this problem, merely calls another aide and asks her to work a double shift to cover the absence. While this solution takes care of the situation for the moment, it does not deal with the real problem. The nurse-manager has not explored the reasons for the predictable absence. In addition, the consequences of the chosen alternative have not been explored. The criteria used for selecting the chosen alternative are vague and perhaps faulty. The eventual consequences of nurse-manager behavior of this type is staff dissatisfaction and a potential increase in absenteeism. An even more severe potential consequence of this solution is that the quality of client care can decrease due to the decrease in energy level of persons assuming additional work assignments. In essence, the nurse-manager provides an easy solution to the immediate problem while the real problem is ignored. This type of problem solving is likened to putting a finger in the hole of a dike. As soon as the finger is removed, the problem is back.

The nurse-manager who uses creativity in solving recurring problems will act in yet another way. Periodically, the persistent problems are reviewed and deliberate investigation of the problems is scheduled. Noting the month's absences, the nurse-manager schedules a creative problem-solving session with the staff. The meeting includes the persons who are causing the problem. The nurse-manager begins the meeting by identifying the fuzzy problem area and writing it on the chalkboard. It reads:

EXAMPLE

Frequent Friday Absences

The nurse-manager begins the session by providing the staff with facts.

1) Each Friday this month, one aide called in sick.
2) Each time this occurred, the next two days were regularly scheduled days off for the person.
3) Each time this happened it was necessary for another aide to work an extra shift.

4) The aide, calling in sick, was paid for the day off duty.

5) The aide covering the absence was paid time and a half for overtime work.

6) The financial cost to the agency was, therefore, $1\frac{1}{2}$ times more than ordinary for that eight hour shift.

7) On two occasions it took three telephone calls to get someone else to cover.

8) The director of nursing is concerned about the situation.

After presenting the original list of facts, the group is asked to brainstorm the problem, deferring judgment. The following list of ideas emerge from that session:

1) Dock the worker.

2) Have the worker get a doctor's note confirming illness.

3) Have the worker work on Sunday to cover.

4) Do not give her her next scheduled weekend.

5) Have her get her own replacement.

6) Have her call the director of nurses and explain the absence.

7) Make her cover for the person that covered for her.

8) Record it on her evaluation.

9) No merit raises for persons doing this.

*10) Pay employees for unused sick time at the end of the year.

*11) Give periodic three day weekends

*12) Change to 10 hour day, four day work week

13) Fire aides and replace with professional staff

14) Give series of lectures on responsibilities of workers

15) Terminate contracts

16) Hire a consultant to study the problem

17) Transfer the worker to another unit

18) Transfer the worker to night shift

19) Publish in agency newspaper the names of persons absent from work

20) Ask absent persons to determine their own penalties

The nurse-manager then explains to the group that the intent of the session is not to be punitive. The desire is to see if a rational solution can be found for dealing with the problem. She/he asks the group to look over the list and see which ideas have the most potential for providing a solution to the problem. The group selected numbers 10, 11 and 12 (indicated with *).

These ideas are rephrased in creative format and now read:

1) How might we pay employees for unused sick time at the end of the year?

2) How might we give periodic three day weekends?

3) How might we change to 10 hour day, four day work weeks?

The nurse-manager calls to the groups' attention that the fuzzy problem is now changed dramatically. He/she asks the group if they are sure that the three problems which now appear on the chalkboard are ones that they want to explore further. The group agrees to the new statements of the problem.

DISCUSSION

It should be noted that the original solution used by the nurse-manager did not come close to solving the real problem. It now seems to indicate that the aides want more concentrated time off duty and want to be compensated for sick time that they do not use. These issues were at the core of the problem but were not explored by using the finger in the dike method of decision making. Restating the problems in this format makes it possible to be futuristic and allows the potential for decreasing absenteeism rather than coping with the results of absenteeism.

The nurse-manager explains to the group that the criteria used to assess the alternatives generated to solve the problem will be:

1) staff satisfaction
2) feasibility
3) cost
4) long-range effects on organization
5) short-range effects on organization

The nurse-manager deliberately exposes the group to the assessment criteria so they have a better understanding of how decisions are made. This position allow the staff to grow and to take part in the entire decision-making process.

Decision Making Regarding Staff Turnover

The staff turnover is unusually high and the nurse manager is deeply concerned that the remaining staff members will become overworked and also resign. A meeting is scheduled to use the five step creative problem-solving process—fact-finding, problem-finding, idea-finding, solution-finding, and acceptance-finding—to investigate staffing problems.

The following example is the result of the group problem solving.

EXAMPLE

FUZZY PROBLEM:

How to improve staffing.

MESS:

Hospital seems understaffed. Staff turnover is high, morale is low.

FACT FINDING:

two month delay for float nurses to receive salaries

16 bed units filled to capacity

$4.00 per month for parking but no guaranteed space

no child care services

starting salary $1000 per month

below $12,000 per year receive 6% raise

above $12,000 per year receive 3% raise

four blocks to walk from parking

pay $15.00 towards Blue Cross and Blue Shield

one registered nurse per each eight hours

one licensed vocational nurse per each eight hours

social security paid by agency

increase in salary due to social security will be taxed

20% of hospital in-patient fees paid

approval is needed for compensation time (overtime)

The group wanted answers to the following areas to clarify the facts:

What types of merit raises are available?

What are the overtime expectations?

How many shifts (rotating) are staff nurses working?

What is the nurse-patient ratio?

What is the difference in salary between this agency and neighboring agencies?

What is the differential salary for evenings, nights, and holidays?

What is the paid vacation time?

What is paid towards tuition for additional education?

What is the leave time policy for additional education and meetings?

What is the length of the orientation program?

Who decides which staff nurses will attend continuing education offerings?

PROBLEM-FINDING:

The following creative statements emerged from the fact-finding session:

In what ways might I (we)

— help to solve the staffing problems?

— improve fringe benefits to staff nurses?

— increase interest in in-service education?

— increase educational offerings to staff nurses?

— prevent resignations?

— increase the level of preparation of ancillary personnel?

— increase the nurse to patient ratio?

— increase health team collaboration?

— decrease the number of times nurses are "floated" to other areas?

— decrease the overtime expectations?

— improve the parking situation?

— get child care facilities?

— provide coverage for meals away from the unit?

— make coffee breaks operational?

— decrease nonnursing functions from the nurses' work load?

— get differential salary for increased educational preparation?

— increase collaboration between the hospital staff and the University School of Nursing?

— increase salaries?

— increase communication between nursing and other hospital departments?

— provide preparation to staff and head nurses related to management?

It was obvious that many subproblems resulted from the original problem statement. The group decided that parking was a major concern and decided to take this subproblem to problem solve first.

IDEA-FINDING:

In what ways might I (we) improve the parking situation for staff nurses and ancillary nursing personnel?

The brainstorming session, using deferred judgment, resulted in the following list of ideas:

 *1) Make it free.
  2) Make it closer.
  3) Mini train.
 *4) Guards to accompany nurses to their cars during dark periods.
 *5) Lighted areas.
  6) Covered parking.
 *7) Covered ramps between parking and hospital.
  8) Move.
  9) Guaranteed spaces.
 10) Car pools.
 11) Park and ride.
 12) Compact car spots.
 13) Underground tunnels.

14) 24 hour gas station.
15) Service man.
16) Protection for bikes.
17) Additional buses.
18) Delivery to home.
19) Train from Houston.
20) Train from Pasadena.
21) Bus from Houston.
22) Vans from Houston.
23) Vans with educational programs.
*24) Car pool vans.
25) Boats.
26) Lockers.
27) Helicopter.
28) Patrol guards in parking areas.
29) Bicycle racks.

The brainstorming period ended with numbers 1, 4, 5, 7, 24, and 28 (indicated by *) as the most promising alternatives.

SOLUTION-FINDING:

The criteria chosen to evaluate the ideas were cost, time, and feasibility. The table on page 162 reflects the group's evaluation based on a scale of one to three with one being the lowest score and three being the most probable.

The escort guards receive the highest rating while the lighted areas, patrol guards, and vans for car pooling were worthy of consideration as alternatives.

ACCEPTANCE-FINDING:

The group decided that rejection of their ideas was the worst thing that might happen to their request for escort guards to accompany nurses to their cars during nondaylight hours. They decided to do the following to help decrease the probability that their suggestion would be rejected:

1) Get 15 nurses to sign a petition to lend support to the idea.
2) Make an appointment with the supervisor of the security guards and get his input.
3) Talk to the assistant hospital administrator and the director of nurses about the idea.
4) Seek legal council.

After completing the list of "to do's" they established this timetable:

1) within two weeks.
2) within three weeks.
3) within three weeks.
4) within two weeks.

IDEAS	COST	TIME	FEASIBILITY	TOTAL
Covered walkways	1	1	1	3
Free parking	1	1	2-3	4-5
Lighted parking areas	1-2	2	3	6-7
Patrol guards	1	2	3	6
Vans—car pooling	0	3	2-3	5-6
Escort guards	2	2	3	7 *

DISCUSSION

During the process of nurturing creativity, the participants are made aware of the vast amount of data available to use in a variety of ways in the decision-making process. A major goal is to broaden the base from which decisions are made by including more data and varied viewpoints in the deliberations. This broadened base results in the generation of additional alternatives which leads to the probability of increasing the acceptability of the decisions that are made. When too few alternatives are available, the tendency is to copy established alternatives whether or not they are successful in solving the problem. Decisions made on the basis of this precedence tend to perpetuate discontent rather than dissolve or lessen it.

Nursing Rounds and Reports

The nursing manager makes rounds with the staff on the unit to determine the health status of the clients. In the course of the rounds, the staff is requested to identify the problems of each client and the solutions proposed for approaching the problems. The problem-solving process is encouraged by the nurse-manager asking, "What else might be done?" "Who else might help?" "Why is it important?" "What else would you like to do?" "What do the clients' significant others think about the situation?" Each of these questions has the potential for purging the minds of the staff members. The nurse-manager who involves the staff in rounds which focus on generating ideas rather than giving information is helping the staff to learn to work through client situations in a creative manner. At the end of the day, the report to personnel on the next shift focuses on the present status of the problem solving in relation to each client. Difficult situations can be problem solved by the personnel of both shifts to increase the input into the problem resolution.

The nurse-manager is appraised of clients having special problems which do not respond to the alternatives generated by the personnel. This information is presented in written format. This report serves as the basis for the nurse-manager's report to his/her supervisor.

The aims of rounds and written reports are to highlight the creative thinking expended on behalf of clients and to stimulate further thinking about ways to facilitate quality care for each of the clients on the nursing unit. Reports and rounds help to motivate the staff members to work collaboratively with clients and each other to resolve client, unit, and staffing problems. In a milieu that is dedicated to helping clients and staff members realize their fullest potential, there is less possibility for disagreements to arise regarding the best course of action as everyone is involved in finding the most suitable alternatives and implementing them.

Motivation of Employees

Genius is one percent inspiration and ninety-nine percent perspiration.

Thomas Alva Edison

The nurse manager realizes that one of the most challenging parts of the role is to motivate staff members to do the best job possible. In order to motivate persons, it is necessary to identify means to help staff members internalize the need to do an excellent job, or a better job, or an additional job. The employee is not always motivated by the same reasons or rewards as perceived by the nurse-manager to be successful motivation stimulators.

The nurse manager begins the process of motivation by extolling an enthusiasm for high quality client care. The manager's pride in nursing, as a profession, goes a long way in instilling a sense of pride in coworkers. In addition, the self-pride generated by providing quality care to clients is a reinforcer and motivator for the employee. The nurse manager must be astute to reinforce the self-pride displayed by employees. Acknowledging quality nursing care and rewarding employees on the basis of it will go a long way in serving as a motivator to encourage future professional excellence. There should be no doubt within the organizational structure that employees are rewarded for the quality of care they render on behalf of clients. If there is any doubt that this is the case, the probability that rewards will be motivators to assure quality client care is decreased.

Another way to motivate staff members is to set high standards for quality nursing care and to uphold them. The staff member is kept appraised of how his/her performance differs from the anticipated standards of care established for the agency. This focus on the discrepancy between acceptable standards of care, and the actual performance of the employee can serve as a motivational force for improving performance. It must be quite clear to the employee that the standards of care will not be lowered, therefore his/her performance must be improved to reach the established standard. Conferences between nurse managers and employees which focus on the expected level of performance and observed discrepancies help the employee to know where improvement is proposed and to set a timetable for achieving the goal. In addition, the limits which will be tolerated until the goal is achieved are identified and made clear to the employee so there is no possibility that the employee is unclear about the expectations. It is best to put the information in writing to try to limit the amount of misunderstanding that can occur when nurse-manager-employee evaluative conferences are held.

Inherent in the need to motivate employees is the need to provide ongoing educational opportunities for employees to update their knowledge and skills. The process of knowledge acquisition is partially based on making connections between known facts and facts which need to be acquired. Memory is the process of linking and making associations or connections with past learned material. The more knowledge that is stored for retrieval, the easier it is for the person to learn new material which is closely related to the stored material.

The nurse-manager, as facilitator of learning, can use exercises which require employees to make these connections through the use of exercises similar to the ones that follow:

EXERCISES AND DISCUSSION

EXERCISE 1: DISCREPANCY LEARNING

Robert is 27 years old. He has just been placed on peritoneal dialysis. This is done to rid the body of wastes. Please write down as many ideas as you can to the following three questions.

How is peritoneal dialysis similar to coffee perked through a filter paper?
How are they alike?
How are they unlike?

DISCUSSION:

The nurse-manager is utilizing a well-known concept related to perking coffee to try to make an unknown situation seem less threatening to the employees. By asking them to write down how one filtering process compares to another filtering process, the nurse-manager is trying to bridge the gap between the known and the unknown. After each participant works independently, the nurse-manager asks the participants to share their ideas with the group. The sharing of ideas tends to stimulate further thinking.

EXERCISE 2: ANALOGUE AND INDIVIDUAL CONNECTIONS

Mary is six months old and is receiving intravenous feedings. The feedings and equipment vary from the adult requirements. Please write down as many ideas as you can for each of the three questions that follow:

What do you know about the intravenous fluid and equipment requirements of adults?

How is that information *like* the requirements for children?

How is it *unlike* the requirements for children?

DISCUSSION

The nurse-manager continues to use written exercises followed by a sharing of ideas to promote and extend the knowledge base of employees. The emphasis in this exercise is on creative as opposed to logical or critical thinking.

EXERCISE 3: LEARNING RELEVANCY

Please write your answers to the following questions.

What in your experience is like receiving intravenous fluids?

How is it like?

How is it unlike?

DISCUSSION:

In this exercise, the participant is allowed more flexibility in thinking as the nurse manager does not select the comparable situation. This exercise allows for a wider range of responses and usually the responses include feeling states which are seldom included in the two previous exercises.

Again, the participants are invited to share their ideas with the group. Connections with Exercise 3 and the previous exercises are pointed out by the nurse-manager at the end of the discussion period.

In addition, any exercise or practice that tends to dissolve or disrupt fixed associations, stored in the person's conscious or unconscious mind, can serve as stimuli to creativity. The goal of the exercise is to change associations so that they are *novel* rather than literal or conventional. Making novel associations is closely related to the act of creation, expressing creativity, and solving problems creatively.

Encouraging Publishing

The nurse-manager makes it quite clear that creativity in the delivery of nursing services is expected and appreciated. A way to emphasize the value of creativity is to have a nursing conference to feature and share creative approaches to care. In addition, these examples can be shared through agency publications. The nurse-manager encourages employees to submit articles for publication in nursing journals documenting creative approaches to client care. Another approach is to have the local newspaper interview an employee and write an article on the employee's accomplishments. The sharing of creative approaches to the delivery of nursing care is vital to the nursing profession. The profession cannot leave its most creative achievements without extensive visability in its publications. The nurse-manager encourages employees to share their achievements with the entire profession.

Many employees have the idea that they cannot write. This attitude interferes with their motivation to try to write. The nurse-manager attempts to help the staff members overcome their feelings of inferiority or hesitancy in relation to writing. One way to do this is by starting to encourage writing that is not work related to assist them to acquire the "feel" of writing. The exercises on page 72 can be used to stimulate the staff members to do creative writing which will help them to become at ease with writing. After these exercises are completed, the nurse-manager can encourage the employees to write all their ideas about their creative nursing activity in a freewheeling manner, deferring judgment. When all the ideas are down, the article is put aside to allow for incubation to occur. The employee is encouraged to keep a pad and pencil handy so that any ideas which come to mind can be jotted down immediately. A few days later, the original article and all the additional ideas are brought together, and work is started to refine the article. After this is done, the nurse-manager reads the article and offers suggestions and encouragement. Other staff members are invited to read the article and offer suggestions. The review of the article is an attempt to generate additional ideas and for the employee to benefit from positive critique. The employee is encouraged to polish the article and set a timetable for having it ready to submit for consideration for publication. The excitement generated by seeing ideas in print is a strong motivator for doing additional writing. The goal of the nurse-manager is to provide timely assistance to employees to help them to the point where creative accomplishments are shared and used to facilitate the nursing profession's coming of age.

To date, nurse-managers have not been very instrumental in helping their employees become prolific writers. This stance has resulted in the nursing journals being less practice-oriented than journals in many other professions. The true test of a profession is to have its ideas open to scrutiny from others. Nursing practitioners must be encouraged to assume the role of writer if the profession is to benefit substantially from creative ideas. Nurse-managers serve as role models and facilitators of this function.

Creating Change

Change is inevitable in a progressive country. Change is constant.

Benjamin Disraeli

A recurring sign of a creative person is the ability to visualize images in a variety of ways and to devise new combinations of ideas or things to result in a creative outcome. The nurse manager, interested in creating change, must find ways to combine ideas, see new relationships, make unlikely combinations, and force new relationships so she/he can sense new solutions to old problems and create refreshing change. The dilemma comes when the refreshing change is seen as a threat by coworkers. Initially, new ideas tend to have more negative than positive repercussions from colleagues unless the developer is cautious about the way the ideas are introduced and implemented. The nurse-manager is sensitive to the interpretation that some staff members tend to place on new ideas. New ideas can be threatening. Creative people need to temper their own enthusiasm for their ideas until they have the opportunity to help others see the value in the idea and internalize its value.

One of the greatest pains in human nature is the pain of a new idea.

Walter Bagehot

Timing is very important for acceptance of creative ideas. I vividly recall the time when a decision was made to use paper diapers on a pediatric unit. The parents were adamant that they did not want their children clothed in paper diapers. The decision to use paper diapers was based on the persistent shortage of diapers on the pediatric unit due to pilferage combined with laundry turn around time problems. The paper diapers had to be discontinued based on the parent's dissatisfaction with them. By witnessing today's extensive use of disposable diapers one can appreciate the importance of timing for the acceptance or rejection of creative ideas!

The greatest emphasis in the creative problem-solving process, when change is the goal, is on the solution-finding and acceptance-finding stages of the process. This emphasis is paramount if the nurse-manager's role is to go beyond the phase of merely seeking innovative ideas to derive personal satisfaction.

Alex Osborn

The acceptance-finding stage focuses attention on the following: 1) all the persons who will be involved if the idea is implemented; 2) what the benefits will be; 3) any trade-offs from the implementation; 4) the worst thing(s) that could happen if the idea is presented for consideration; 5) what persons would be helpful in getting it implemented; 6) what persons would tend to lose something if the idea is implemented; 7) how much time is needed to achieve the goal; 8) what resources are needed and/or available to help with the project; and 9) a timetable proposed with the most optimistic and pessimistic times for completing the implementation.

The nurse-manager needs to spend considerable time ideating on each of these areas. Time is spent resolving issues before they arise or finding acceptable answers for questions that are raised by persons who will be influenced by the decision. The period of time spent in the acceptance-finding phase is well justified when taking into consideration that it may make the difference between an idea being accepted or rejected. The nurse-manager who takes this phase too lightly is likely to have more ideas rejected than the nurse-manager who considers this phase of problem solving to be just as important as the idea-finding phase. An illustration follows.

EXAMPLE

A sales representative comes to the hospital and demonstrates a new bed for clients with back injuries. The staff members and nurse-manager view the demonstration of the product. The staff members have some reservations about the equipment but leave the room without voicing their concerns. The nurse-manager interprets their silence as satisfaction with the equipment. The decision is made to purchase the new bed. The first time a client with a back injury is admitted, the dissatisfactions with the equipment are raised. The staff members insist they were not involved in the decision to purchase the equipment. They request that the client use the equipment that was used in the past. In order to serve the client's immediate needs, the new equipment has to be put aside and the old bed is used.

DISCUSSION

In this illustration, the solution-finding and acceptance-finding steps in the problem-solving process were not given adequate consideration. The purchase of the equipment was a premature act. Now the nurse-manager is faced with trying to convince the staff members that the decision to purchase the new equipment is the only acceptable idea. It will take more time to resolve the resistance to the change because the staff members do not feel they had a role in deciding the change. An illustration of a better approach follows.

EXAMPLE

The nurse-manager assumes a more active role in the demonstration. After the salesman demonstrates the equipment, the nurse-manager asks the staff members, "What do you like about the equipment?" "What do you dislike about the equipment?" "How is it like our present equipment?" "How is it different?" "Why would you like to have this equipment?" "Why would you not like to have this equipment?" "Do you have any reservations about the equipment?" "If you had to decide whether or not to purchase the equipment, how would you vote?"

The nurse-manager also talks to individual staff members a week later to get impressions after time has elapsed and incubation has taken place. At this time, the nurse-manager is searching for congruence or noncongruence with the original responses of the staff members. Special attention is placed on talking to persons who did not voice their opinions in the demonstration meeting, as a salesperson can be a deterrent to open expression of negative feelings. If incongruence is found, further exploration is needed. The nurse-manager asks, "What additional thoughts did you have to help you change your position?" "Would you like to discuss your concerns with other members of the staff?" "Do you know of equipment we might explore?" "Are you interested in seeing demonstrations of other equipment?"

Based on the feedback from these contacts, it may be necessary to have another staff meeting. If the position to purchase or not to purchase is clear, the decision can be made without another meeting.

If the decision is to purchase the equipment (the idea for a solution), then the nurse-manager focuses attention on the acceptance-finding strategies. The staff members are likely to be more supportive since they were involved in the decision. However, it is still necessary to consider all the things which require attention to smoothly implement the idea. It is wise to plan in-service sessions for the staff members to practice using the equipment in a simulated situation. A timetable for starting and completing these sessions is developed. The staff members sign up to attend the session of their choice. Paraprofessionals from other departments are invited to the simulated experiences so they can become familiar with the new equipment. Letters are sent to schools of nursing who have students in the agency announcing the incorporation of the equipment and asking if they desire to have their faculty and students attend a simulated session. Physicians are notified of the equipment and invited to attend a simulated session. It may be necessary to have housekeeping or maintenance plan special sessions for their staff members. Volunteer persons may need an orientation. The nurse-manager attempts to maintain liaison with these groups so they can plan the necessary action on behalf of their personnel.

The nurse manager heralds the opportunity to create change by deliberately using processes for expanding his/her ways of addressing problems. The following exercises are used to encourage creativity for creating change.

EXERCISES AND DISCUSSION

EXERCISE 1:

Examine a spoon very carefully and then list 15 nonconventional uses for the spoon.

DISCUSSION:

An attempt is made to see articles in a different perspective. The nurse manager is directed to spend a great deal of time focusing on the spoon with the definite intent to see it differently. Stating a definite number of ideas to generate encourages the participant to produce the requested number of ideas.

EXERCISE 2:

Examine a pencil very carefully and then list 15 ways you can change the pencil.

DISCUSSION:

The goal of this exercise is very similar to the previous one. Exercise 1 requires a change by putting the spoon to other uses while this exercise requires the object to change its usual form. Both of these exercises will demonstrate that change is not always difficult, especially if we free ourselves of constraints which bind us to traditional thinking.

Change involves a consideration of questions that concern WHAT-IF statements. The nurse manager asks *what* will happen if I do certain things or if I suggest certain alternatives to the staff. The following exercises are what-if activities.

EXERCISE 1:

What would happen if you could hire and fire all the staff you would like to?

EXERCISE 2:

What would happen if a cure was found for cancer?

EXERCISE 3:

What would happen if National Health Insurance becomes a reality?

EXERCISE 4:

What would happen if elective surgery was disallowed by the federal government?

EXERCISE 5:

What would happen if nurses were replaced by robots?

DISCUSSION:

The what-if questions help to stimulate the imagination. They are another technique for breaking habits and unleashing creative ideas. They are intended to allow the participant to fantasize and generate wild, as well as usual, ideas. The freewheeling thinking process is encouraged in these activities.

The nurse-manager is faced with many situations that require immediate decisions. The following exercises will help to develop skill in this vital area. Try to find six alternatives to resolve each of the situations.

EXERCISE 1:

The emergency room is staffed by one registered nurse and a male attendant. Tuesday afternoon is usually a time when only occasional minor illnesses are treated. Today, an oil rig turns over and 28 men are seriously injured. What ideas can you generate for coping with the situation?

EXERCISE 2:

You are waiting on the fifth floor for the service elevator to bring emergency equipment to the third floor. The four wheeled cart is piled high with supplies. When the elevator arrives, it is filled with people and there is only room for you to get on. What will you do? Generate as many alternatives as you can for resolving this dilemma.

EXERCISE 3:

You have just finished scrubbing your hands to enter the newborn nursery. Your hands are sensitive. The telephone rings and you are the only one in the immediate area. How will you deal with the ringing phone?

EXERCISE 4:

You are covering six floors on a busy weekend. The paging system is not working. How will you keep in touch with the staff on each of the units?

EXERCISE 5:

A philanthropic individual comes to the hospital and gives you gifts to circulate to the administrative staff for being "nice" to his wife who is hospitalized on the third floor where the staffing is low. What will you do?

EXERCISE 6:

The adolescent unit is bombarded with six late admissions. The dietary service is closed until morning. All six of the adolescents are groaning from hunger pains. They all can eat if you can find the food. What will you do?

EXERCISE 7:

Visiting hours end at ten each evening. The security department is eager to have all visitors out of the building by 10:30 P.M. As the administrative officer on evenings, the chief of security calls you to voice his concerns about the visitors who repeatedly ignore the policy. What will you do to help alleviate this problem?

DISCUSSION:

In crisis situations it is necessary to be resourceful in order to function effectively in the system. Resourcefulness is the act of being creative in finding alternatives for life's challenges.

Conclusion

The role of the nurse-manager is somewhat ill-defined. The nurse-manager is involved in a variety of experiences that relate to "managing" a system of diversified employees. If definite attempts are not made to the contrary, the role can lead to a structured nondemocratic system of interaction. The use of creativity, combined with logical thinking, is a viable alternative for facilitating involvement of the employees in the managerial process. The nurse manager has a vital role in the provision of quality health services to clients. Therefore, it is important that the nurse-manager use all of the problem-solving skills available for guaranteeing that quality services will be given.

References

Chapter 1

1. Osborn AE: Applied Imagination, ed 3. New York, Charles Scribner's Sons, 1963, p 1.
2. DeBono E: Lateral Thinking: Creativity Step by Step. New York, Harper & Row Publishers, 1973.
3. DeBono E: PO: A Device for Successful Thinking. New York, Simon & Schuster, 1972.
4. Verne J: Twenty Thousand Leagues Under the Sea. New York, Charles Scribner's Sons, 1925.
5. Hilgard ER, Atkinson RC, Atkinson RL: Introduction to Psychology, ed 6. New York, Harcourt, Brace, Jovanovich Inc, 1975, pp 151-157.

Chapter 2

1. Sperry RW: Perception in the absence of neocortical commissures, in Perception and its disorders. Proceedings of the Association for Research in Nervous and Mental Disease 48:1968.

Chapter 3

1. Schneider L: Be Careful of What You Want, You Might Get It. Roanoke, Virginia, Stone Printing Co, 1970.
2. Mooney RL: Lecture-demonstration on perception as a transaction, prepared for advanced students in education. Columbus, Ohio, Visual Demonstration Center, 1951.

Chapter 4

1. Guilford JP: Factors that aid and hinder creativity, in Dauw DC, Fredian AJ(eds): Creativity and Innovation in Organizations. Dubuque, Iowa, Kendall/Hunt Publishing Co, 1971, pp 75-95.

Chapter 5

1. Crawford RP: The Techniques of Creative Thinking: How to Use Your Ideas to Achieve Success. New York, Hawthorn Books, 1954.
2. Osborn AF: Applied Imagination, ed 3. New York, Charles Scribner's Sons, 1963, p 151.
3. Gildersleeve T: So you'd like to be more creative. Data Management 13:31-35, 1975.
4. Mackenzie E: Managing creative people. International Management 25:56-68, 1970.
5. Steiner GA: The Creative Organization. Chicago, Univ Chicago Press, 1965, pp 258-259.

Chapter 6

1. Koprowski E: Creativity, Man and Organizations. J Creative Behavior 1:49-54, 1972.
2. Cummings L: Organizational Climates for Creativity, in Chruden HJ, Sherman AW: Readings in Personnel Management, ed 4. Cincinnati, Ohio, South-Western Pub Co, 1976, pp 220-227, 226.
3. Gildersleeve T: So you'd like to be more creative. Data Management 13:31-35, 1975.
4. MacKenzie E: Managing creative people. International Management 25:56-68, 1970.
5. Steiner GA: The Creative Organization. Chicago, Univ Chicago Press, 1965, pp 258-259.

Chapter 7

1. Osborn AF: Applied Imagination. New York, Charles Scribner's Son, 1963.
2. Parnes SJ, Noller RB, Biondi AM: Guide to Creative Action. New York, Charles Scribner's Sons, 1976.
3. Eberle RF: Scamper. Buffalo, New York, DOK Pub, 1971.

Chapter 8

1. Maslow AH: Toward a Psychology of Being, ed. 2. New York, Van Nostrand Rheinhold, 1968.
2. Zinker J: Creative Process in Gestalt Therapy. New York, Vintage Books, 1977.
3. Martindale C: What makes creative people different. Psychol Today 9:44, 1975.
4. Moustakas C: Creativity and Conformity. New York. D Van Nostrand Co, 1967.
5. DiCyan E: Creativity: Road to Self-Discovery. New York, Jove Pub, 1978.

Chapter 9

1. MacKinnon DW: In Search of Human Effectiveness. New York, Creative Synergetic Assoc, 1978.
2. Zinker J: Creative Process in Gestalt Therapy. New York, Vintage Books, 1977.
3. Maslow AH: The Farther Reaches of Human Nature. New York, Penguin Books, 1971.
4. Moustakes C: Creativity and Conformity. New York, D Van Nostrand Co, 1967.
5. May R: The Courage to Create. New York, Bantam Books, 1975.
6. Moustakas CE: Loneliness and Love. New Jersey, Prentice-Hall, 1972.
7. Martindale C: What makes creative people different. Psychol Today 9:44, 1975.
8. Merton T: Contemplation in a World of Action. New York, Image Books, 1973, pp 178, 179.
9. Stevens JO: Awareness: Exploring Experimenting Experiencing, New York, Bantam Books, 1971.
10. Heintz AC, Fieweger M, Fitzgerald P: Independent Learning. Lexington, Mass, Ginn Co, 1975.
11. Flach FF: Choices. Philadelphia, JB Lippincott Co, 1977.
12. Broudy HS: Arts education: necessary or just nice? Phi Delta Kappa 60:347-350, 1979.
13. Maslow AH: Toward a Psychology of Being, ed 2. New York, Van Nostrand Rheinhold, 1968.
14. DiCyan E: Creativity: Road to Self-Discovery. New York, Jove Pub, 1978.
15. Steele S, Maraviglia F: Creative Problem-Solving in Nursing Workshop. Galveston, Texas School of Nursing at Galveston, August 23, 25, 1978.

Chapter 10

1. Schlotfeldt R: Knowledge, leaders and progress. Image 2:5, 1978.
2. Ackoff RL: The Art of Problem Solving. New York, John Wiley & Sons, 1968.
3. Morris W (ed): The American Heritage Dictionary. Boston, Houghton Mifflin Co, 1976.
4. Pfeiffer JW, Jones J: A Program for Getting Acquainted in Depth. LaJolla, California, University Assoc, 1974.
5. MacKinnon DW: In Search of Human Effectiveness. New York, Creative Synergetic Assoc, 1978.
6. Flanders NA: Interaction Models of Critical Teaching Behaviors, in Armidon EJ, Hough JB (ed): Interaction Analysis: Theory, Research and Application. Massachusetts, Addison-Wesley Pub, 1967, pp 371-402.
7. Hough JB, Duncan JK: Teaching: Description and Analysis. Massachusetts, Addison-Wesley Pub, 1970.
8. Pearson BD: Use of the Five Senses in Acquiring Professional Skills. Nursing Reseach 23:259-262, 1974.
9. Parnes S: 24th Annual Creative Problem Solving Workshop. Buffalo, New York, 1978.
10. Heintz AC, Fieweger M, Fitzgerald P: Independent Learning. Lexington, Massachusetts, Ginn & Co, 1975, p 51.
11. Lynch D (ed): Teleido-letter 1:7, 1978.

Chapter 11

1. Moustakas C: Creativity and Conformity. New York, D Van Nostrand Co, 1967.
2. Broudy HS: Arts education: Necessary or just nice? Phi Delta Kappa 60:347-350, 1979.
3. Goodland JI: Can Our Schools Get Better? Phi Delta Kappa 60:342-347, 1979.
4. Moustakas CE: Loneliness and Love. New Jersey, Prentice-Hall, 1972.
5. MacKinnon DW: In Search of Human Effectiveness. New York, Creative Synergetic Assoc, 1978.
6. Heintz AC, Fieweger M, Fitzgerald P: Independent Learning. Lexington, Massachusetts, Ginn & Co, 1975.
7. Rosen R: Do we really need ends to justify the means? Center Report 7:29-30, 1974.
8. White J: The Highest State of Consciousness. New York, Anchor Books, 1972.

Chapter 12

1. Moustakas C: Creativity and Conformity. New York, D Van Nostrand, Co, 1967.
2. Moustakas CE: Loneliness and Love. New Jersey, Prentice-Hall, 1972.
3. Zinker J: Creative Process in Gestalt Therapy. New York, Vintage Books, 1977.

Chapter 13

1. Ackoff RL: The Art of Problem Solving. New York, John Wiley & Sons, 1968.
2. Psychegenics Newsletter. Gaithersburg, Maryland, Winter 1978.
3. MacKinnon DW: In Search of Human Effectiveness. New York, Creative Synergetic Assoc, 1978.
4. DiCyan E: Creativity: Road to Self-Discovery. New York, Jove Pub, 1978.
5. Stevens BJ: First-Line Patient Care Management. Massachusetts, Contemporary Pub Inc, 1976.

Bibliography

Part I

Barrett FD: Creativity techniques: yesterday, today and tomorrow. SAK Advanced Management Journal 43:25-35, 1978.

Bartow PE: Brainstorming. Management Review 64:54-58, 1975.

Boettinger H: Is management really an art? Harvard Business Review 53:54-64, 1975.

Breton EJ: Cultivating and inducing inventions. Research Management 18:19-23, 1975.

Byrd RE: Daring to be different. Industry Week 185:29-34, 1975.

Cummings L: Organizational climates for creativity, in Readings In Personnel Management, ed 4. Cincinnati, Ohio, South-Western Pub Co, 1976, pp 220-227.

Cummings L, Hinton BL, Gobdel BC: Creative behavior as a function of task environment: Impact of objectives, procedures and controls. J Academy Management 18:488-499, 1975.

Delias M, Gaier EL: Identification of the creative in the individual. Psychol Bull 73:55-73, 1970.

Donnelly JF: Participative management at work. Harvard Business Review 55:117-127, 1977.

Edwards MO: Creativity solves management problems. J Systems Management 26:14-20, 1975.

Eschenfelder AH: Positive steps that nourish both research and technological progress. Research Management 11:231-240, 1968.

Feinberg MR: Fourteen suggestions for managing scientific creativity. Management Review 58:25-29, 1968.

Flowers VS, Hughes CL: Choosing a leadership style. Personnel J 57:48-57, 1978.

Gellerman SW: Supervision: Substance and style. Harvard Business Review 54:89-99, 1976.

Gibb JR: Managing for creativity in the organization, in Taylor CW (ed): Climate For Creativity. New York, Pergamon Press, 1972, pp 23-32.

Gildersleeve T: So you'd like to be more creative. Data Management 13:31-35, 1975.

Guilford JP: Factors that aid and hinder creativity, in Dauw JC, Fredian AL (eds): Creativity and Innovation in Organizations. Dubuque, Iowa, Kendall/Hunt Publishing Co, 1971, pp 75-95.

Gyllenhammer PG: How Volvo adapts work to people. Harvard Business Review 55:102-113, 1977.

Harriman B: Up and down the communications ladder. Harvard Business Review 55:143-151, 1977.

Jants AH: The encouragement of employee creativity and initiative. Personnel J 54:476-477, 1975.

Jones JC: Design Methods: Seeds of Human Futures. London, John Wiley & Sons, 1976.

Kafka VW: Encourage the use of creative energy. Supervisory Management 20:32-35, 1975.

Koprowski EJ: Creativity, man and organizations. J Creative Behavior 1:49-54, 1972.

Kubie LS: Blocks to creativity, in Mooney RL, Razik TA (eds): Explorations in Creativity. New York, Harper & Row, 1967, pp 35-43.

MacKenzie E: Managing creative people. International Management 25:56-58, 1970.

Marsh RJ: Overcoming the habits that block creativity. Machine Design 48:52-56, 1976.

Maslow AH: Emotional blocks to creativity, in Parnes SJ, Harding HF (eds): A Source Book for Creative Thinking. New York, Charles Scribner's Sons, 1962, pp 93-105.

Mintzberg H: The manager's job: Folklore and fact. Harvard Business Review 53:49-61, 1975.

Morley E, Silver A: A film director's approach to managing creativity. Harvard Business Review 55:59-70, 1977.

Patrick JP: Organizational climate and the creative individual, in Chruden HJ, Sherman AW: Readings in Personnel Management, ed 4. Cincinnati, Ohio, South-Western Pub Co, 1976, pp 347-354.

Randall L: Organizational paradox. Harvard Business Review 146:86-87, 1965.

Repucci L: Creating a climate for employee innovation. Management Review 57:55-57, 1968.

Rotondi T: The innovator and the ritualist: A study in conflict. Personnel J 53:439-444, 1974.

Sasser W, Skinner EW: Managers with impact: Versatile and inconsistent. Harvard Business Review 55:140-148, 1977.

Souder WE, Ziegler RW: A review of creativity and creative problem solving techniques. Research Management 20:34-42, 1977.

Steiner GA: The Creative Organization. Chicago, Univ Chicago Press, 1965.

Taylor CW: Can organizations be creative, too? in Taylor CW (ed): Climate for Creativity, New York, Pergamon Press, 1972, pp 23-32.

Torrance EP: Education and creativity, in Taylor CW (ed): Creativity: Progress and Potential, New York, McGraw-Hill Book Co, 1964, pp 98-107.

Tumin M: Obstacles to creativity, in Parnes SJ, Harding HF (eds): A Source Book for Creative Thinking. New York, Charles Scribner's Sons, 1962, pp 105-113.

Watson CE: Developing creative people. Research Management 18:14-18, 1975.

Weiss B: How to manage the creative person. Management Review 63:37-40, 1974.

Whitfield R: Turning ideas to advantage. International Management 31:51-52, 1976.

Williams W: What every worker wants, in Chruden HJ, Sherman HW: Readings In Personnel Management, ed 4. Cincinnati, Ohio. South-Western Pub Co, 1976, pp 22-33.

Zalenik A: Managers and leaders: Are they different? Harvard Business Review. 55:67-78, 1977.

Part II

Anderson NL: An interactive systems approach to problem solving. Nurse Practitioner 3:25-26, 1978.

Bach GR, Goldberg H: Creative Aggression. New York, Avon Books, 1974.

Bailey JT et al: Evaluation of the development of creative behavior in an experimental nursing program. Nurs Res 19:100-108, 1970.

Bowers BH: Promoting creativity in nursing education. Hosp Prog 52:64-65, 1971.

Burgess G: The personal development of the nursing student as a conceptual framework. Nurs Forum 17:96, 1978.

Campbell D: Take the Road to Creativity and Get Off Your Dead End. Niles, Illinois, Argus Communications, 1977.

Corona D: Sedatives and stimulants to creativity. Nurs Outlook 12:24-26, 1964.

Eberle B, Hall RE: Affective Education Guidebook. Buffalo, New York, DOK Pub, 1975.

Eberle RF: Scamper. Buffalo, New York, DOK Pub, 1971.

Fearn L: Individual development: a process model in creativity. J Creative Behavior 10:55-64, 1976.

Fosdick HE: On Being A Real Person. New York, Harper & Row Pub, 1977.

Gardner J: Self-Renewal. New York, Harper & Row Pub, 1963.

Harty MB: Goal oriented creativity. Image 5:7-10, 1973.

Herrscher BR: Implementing Individualized Instruction. Houston, Texas Archem Co, 1971.

Kalisch B: Creativity and nursing research. Nurs Outlook 23:314-319, 1975.

Klug C: Judgment and creative thinking. Image 5:10-15, 1973.

Kramer M, Tegan E, Knauber J: The effect of presents on creative problem solving. Nurs Research 19:303-311, 1970.

Levine ME: On creativity in nursing. Image 5:15-19, 1973.

Mayeroff M: On Caring. New York, Harper & Row Pub, 1971.

Noller RB, Parnes SJ, Biondi AM: Creative Actionbook. New York, Charles Scribner's Sons, 1976.

Osborn AF: Applied Imagination. New York, Charles Scribner's Sons, 1963.

Parnes SJ: CPSI: the general system. J Creative Behavior 11:1-11, 1977.

Partridge KB: Nursing values in a changing society. Nurs Outlook 26:356-360, 1978.

Peplau H: Creativity and commitment in nursing. Image 6:13-15, 1974.

Raudsepp E, Hough GP: Creative Growth Games. New York, Jove Pub, 1977.

Reilly DE: Teaching and evaluating the Affective Domain in Nursing Programs. New Jersey, Charles B Slack Inc, 1978.

Robinson A: Creativity takes courage. Nursing Outlook 11:499-501, 1963.

Schweer JE, Gebbie KM: Creative Teaching in Clinical Nursing. St Louis, CV Mosby, 1976.

Seldes G: The Great Quotations. New Jersey, Castle Books, 1966.

Stevens BJ: The Nurse as Executive. Mass, Contemporary Pub, 1975.

Stevens JO: Awareness: Exploring Experimenting Experiencing. New York, Bantam Books, 1971.

Taylor C: Are we utilizing our creative potentials? Nurs Outlook 11:105-107, 1963.

Torrance PH: Does nursing education reduce creativity? Nurs Outlook 12:27-30, 1964.

Verhonick PJ: Creativity through research at the undergraduate level. Image 5:19-23, 1973.

List of Films and Film Companies

Films

The following list of films can be used in several of the exercises in the text. The list was adapted from a film list handout of the Creative Problem Solving Institute in Buffalo, New York.

A CHAIRY TALE   6 min.

A fairy tale in modern manner, told without words, is a kind of simple ballet of a youth and a common kitchen chair. This young man tries to sit, but the chair declines to be sat upon. The ensuing struggle, first for mastery and then for understanding, forms the story.

International Film Bureau

A DAY IN THE LIFE OF BONNIE CONSOLO   *16-1/2 min.*

Bonnie Consolo is an unusual and inspirational woman born without arms, yet she leads a normal and productive life. The film follows her through a typical day as she cares for her home and family, and as she goes about her daily routine she share her thoughts about life. To Bonnie, the world is a beautiful and wonderous place, and she radiates a rich philosophy that inspires everyone to live life to its fullest.

Barr Films

DOT AND THE LINE   *Color*   *9 min.*

An award-winning animation about a dot and a line. It proceeds to explore two plane geometric relationships in a fascinating and delightful fashion that will make young and old alike more mathematically perceptive.

Films Incorporated

DIMENSIONS   Color   13 min.

An animated "play" on the size of things, where all the customary proportions must be achieved, often with amusing results. Filmed without words, it is essentially a children's film, but all will enjoy its simplicity, charm, witty stop motion special effects, and its message: all things are relevant, even on the comic screen.

Films, Inc.

EGO STATES   30 min.

Program No. 1 from the "Learning to Live" series. Ego States is the term used in TA for the three ways people feel and respond. We all have a Parent, Adult, and Child ego states. This film describes and illustrates the characteristics of each Ego State.
Mass Media, Inc.

FUTURE SHOCK   Color   42 min.

This film, taken from the Alvin Toffler book of the same name, describes the world of tomorrow and the changes people must face in the emerging industrialism of today.
Contemporary/McGraw-Hill Films

IMAGINATION AT WORK   21 min.

By means of a story about a pantomimist who inherits a brick factory, the major barriers to creative thought as well as the factors which contribute to creative ability are explained.
Roundtable Films, Inc.

IS IT ALWAYS RIGHT TO BE RIGHT?   Color   8 min.

Deals with the importance of openness and receptivity—insights into human relations, self-development, communications, and perception.
Roundtable Films, Inc.

THE JOY OF COMMUNICATION   18 min.

Depicts communication between people of all ages showing the reciprocal joy of sharing values and experiences—between young and old, parents and children, teacher and student, including the handicapped.
Dana Productions

KOESTLER ON CREATIVITY   Color   40 min.

Arthur Koestler talks about his goals in writing this film which investigates some of the processes underlying the creative act. "This film is based on the book *The Act of Creation*. Although the main emphasis is on the scientist, not the artist, I have tried to indicate that the conscious and unconscious processes underlying the creative act are based in both cases on much the same pattern."
Time-Life Films, Inc.

TOUCHING   35 min.

This film is a conversation with Dr. Ashley Montagu. Utilizing psychological research and medical opinion, Dr. Montagu develops the case that touching is necessary for human life. He utilizes much

experimental research, including the work of Harry Harlow, and clinical work in various settings to develop his thesis.
Psychological Films, Inc.

UP IS DOWN   Color   6 min.

A commentary on the attempt by the majority to make individuals conform. (Animated cartoon.)
Pyramid Films

VISUAL PERCEPTION   18 min.

Presents the work of Dr. Hadley Cantril, psychologist, at the Perception Demonstration Center at Princeton University, in his study of the effects of some of our assumptions on what we see, and how faulty assumptions may lead to incorrect judgments. Examples used are the distorted room, the rotating trapizoid, and balloons which appear to move.
Kent State University

WHY MAN CREATES   Color   25 min.

This film is a series of explorations, episodes, and comments on creativity. Each segment of the film makes its own statement in its own style and technique.
Pyramid Films

YOU CAN SURPASS YOURSELF   28 min.

Demonstrates the acceptance of a challenge, which if pursued, shows that more is within one's reach than the individual ever allows himself to feel.
Ramic Productions

YOU PACK YOUR OWN CHUTE   Color   30 min.

The concept that an individual can control his own destiny, create his own successes and failures, is explored in human, everyday terms. This is further demonstrated by a woman who puts her thesis to the test by parachuting from a plane 3,000 feet over the Pacific.
Ramic Productions

Film Companies

BarrFilms
P.O. Box 7-C
Pasedena, CA 91104

Dana Productions
6249 Babcock Ave.
North Hollywood, CA 91606

Films, Inc.
1144 Wilmette Ave.
Wilmette, IL 60091

International Film Bureau, Inc.
332 S. Michigan Ave.
Chicago, IL 60604

Kent State University
Audio Visual Services
Kent, OH 44242

Psychological Films
Administrative Office
111 North Wheeler St.
Orange, CA 92669

Pyramid Films
Box 1048
Santa Monica, CA 90406

Ramic Productions Films
60 West 57th St.
New York, NY 10019

Roundtable Films, Inc.
113 North San Vicente Blvd.
Beverly Hill, CA 90211

Time-Life Films, Inc.
Distribution Center
Multimedia Division
100 Eisenhower Drive
Paramus, NJ 07652

List of Records

The following records can be used with several exercises in the text. The list is adapted from catalogues describing the records. Teacher supply stores can order the records if they are not in stock.

EXERCISE IS KID STUFF

Children's Songs for Rhythmic Activities. By Douglas and Gloria Evans.

Objective: To encourage development of rhythm, flexibility, endurance, and coordination while stimulating creativity. Focus: Eleven demonstrative melodies promote interesting exercise sessions. Children perform to Little Ducks, Toot the Flute, Celery Stalks, and others. Accompanying manual is graphically illustrated, contains song lyrics and suggested movements and activities.

LP and Manual. Side 1—vocal and music; Side 2—music only.

Kimbo Record.

GET FIT WHILE YOU SIT

By Ambrose Brazelton and Gabriel DeSantis

Objective: To develop muscle strength, fitness, and coordination.

Focus: Activities are done seated. Talk through and walk through instructions with musical accompaniment enhance listening skills, auditory perception, and aural memory.

LP & Guide

Kimbo Record

PLAYTIME PARACHUTE FUN

By Georgiana Liccione Stewart

Words & Music by Jill Gallina

Objective: To aid in the development of gross motor skills and spatial awareness.

Focus: Using a specially designed small-sized parachute, six feet in diameter, these simplified structured parachute activities are ideal for classrooms and limited spaces. The lightweight parachute is easily managed by young children and children with special needs. Original music and lyrics create an imaginative atmosphere for an unusual motor learning activity.

Selections include: Bumping and Jumping, Parachute Powwow, Parachute Rollerball, Mountain High, Floating Cloud, and others.

LP & Manual

Kimbo Record.

RELAXATION—THE KEY TO LIFE

(A major component of hatha yoga) By Rachelle Goldsmith

Objective: Relaxation is effectively dealt with through the use of instrumental music in combination with the techniques of Jacobson and Sweigard.

Focus: Concentration on the relationship of mind and body, effects of tension on the body, body awareness, and dancing or drawing what one has seen in the mind's eye.

LP & Manual

Kimbal Record.

RHYTHMIC PARACHUTE PLAY

By JoAnn Seker and George Jones

Objective: To develop gross motor skills through rhythmic exercises by utilizing parachute canopies.

Focus: Today's top tunes provide the background for an instructional record aimed at basic parachute activities and group routines, making ripples and waves, an umbrella, a mountain, a mushroom, merry-go-round, and more. Accompanying manual includes suggestions for use and supplementary activities. 2 LPs & Manual, Sides 1 & 2-narration & music; Sides 3 & 4-music only.

Kimbo Records.

SUZY PRUDDEN'S CREATIVE FITNESS FOR CHILDREN

By Suzy Prudden

Objective: To teach children basic motor skills, including muscle development, coordination, and agility while furthering imaginative creativity and enhancing strength.

Focus: A unique and refreshing approach to the fundamentals of warm-up exercises. Two imaginative stories which stress creativity along with movement. The stories have been carefully set to music, which speaks the language of children, encouraging them to learn to move correctly within the structure of a creative learning experience.

LP & Manual

Kimbo Record.

WALK, JOG, RUN

Interval Training for Cardiovascular Fitness by Gabriel J. DeSantis and Lester V. Smith

Objective: To introduce a program which applies interval training principles to obtain the final result of maximal increases in cardiovascular fitness.

Focus: Four, six minute segments of activity music are designed to make individuals feel like moving. Timed rest and work periods insure training without straining. This LP has been arranged so that participants can follow a program based on individual fitness needs. A wide variety of activities can be adapted to the music for both limited and unlimited spaces. A manual with instructions for the development of interval training programs for specific purposes is included. Developed and tested at the Educational Research Council of American in Cleveland, Ohio.

LP & Manual.

Kimbo Record.

WE MOVE TO POETRY

Anthology compiled by Anita Seyler Teacher's Guide by Linda Anderson

Objective: To develop creative movement exploration and poetic awareness and appreciation.

Focus: All poems in this two album series were selected for maximum creative interpretation through movement. The poem is read, followed by a musical interlude in which the child can move. Accompanying Teacher's Guide suggests basic movements.

Kimbo Record.

Creative Problem-Solving Think Book

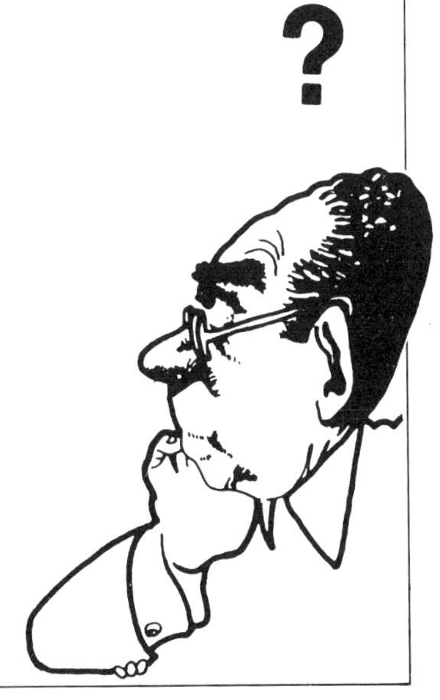

Just make a list of factual* information pertinent to your satisfaction. Circle those facts that you feel are more significant. Who? What? Where? When? Why? How? How often? What about... Texture? Odor? Sound? Taste? Magnitude? Structure? Substance? Color? Shape? Time? Space?

____

____

____

____

____

____

____

____

____

____

____

____

____

____

____

*A fact is a set of data that can be agreed upon. Are there any questions you would like answered?

PROBLEM-FINDING

What do you want to accomplish? What is your objective? Why? Restate your "Situation" from the previous "Fact Finding Worksheet" into questions as follows: (Changing the verb — making it broader or more narrow)

PROBLEMS   FEATURES   BENEFITS

1. In what ways might I . . .

2. In what ways might I . . .

3. In what ways might I . . .

4. In what ways might I . . .

5. In whay ways might I . . .

6. In what ways might I . . .

7. In what ways might I . . .

8. In what ways might I . . .

Now try to pick out what you feel is the real problem, and let's pursue that on the next page.

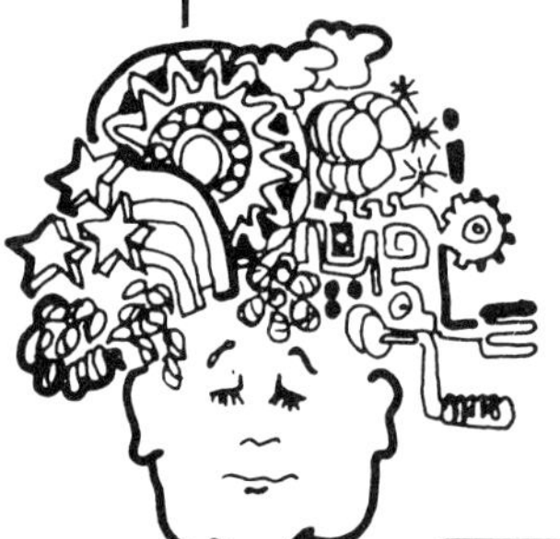

Just make an "option list" (include "unusual ideas", plus practical ideas") Organize; Chain think; Free wheel; Build on and spin off new ideas; (DO NOT JUDGE YET) Use personal and direct analogies; Brainstorm; Incubate; Think metaphorically; Put to other uses; Adapt; Modify; Substitute; Rearrange; Reverse; Combine; Magnify; Minify; How does it feel? What is the paradoxical "Book Title" essence? Algebraic force fit?

Please write your problem finding statement here.

Idea #1.

Idea #2.

Idea #3.

Idea #4.

Idea #5.

Idea #6.

Idea #7.

Idea #8.

Idea #9.

Idea #10.

Idea #11.

Idea #12.

SOLUTION-FINDING

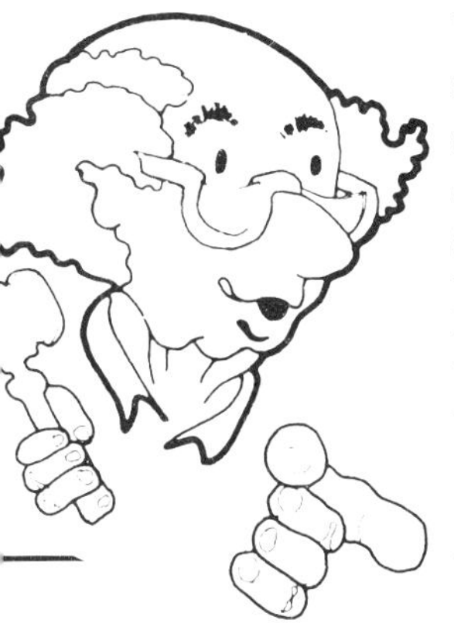

What are the (best, real, critical, tangible) criteria that will measure your ideas in relation to your problem? Score each of your best ideas against the selected criteria, one column at a time. Example scoring scale: 10 = Good, and 0 = Bad. Possible criteria: Cost? Time? Resources? Material? Operating Costs? Capital? Image? Processes? Equipment? Intangible values? Opinions? Attitude? Aesthetics? Chance for success? Safety? Durability? Reliability?

	CRITERIA	CRITERIA	CRITERIA	CRITERIA	TOTAL POINTS

ACCEPTANCE-FINDING

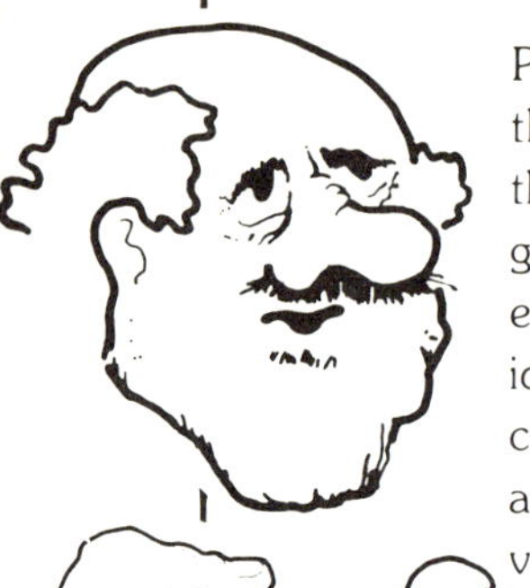

Plan your action — Do your plan. Fantasize and visualize the solution being accepted. How can you share it with those affected? How can it be presented visually or graphically? Who else needs to be sold on the idea? Be enthusiastic. Be persistent, until the adoption of your idea. Be sensitive to the impact on others of social change. Play the devil's advocate and be prepared to answer those objections. Communicate your idea both verbally and non verbally. Know your market.

A. What resources are needed to implement you idea?

1.   3.   5.

2.   4.   6.

B. Who can make those resources available to you?

1.   3.   5.

2.   4.   6.

C. How, when, where, will you pretest, and then apply the resources?	Start Date	Finish Date	Check When Complete

Be enthusiastic. Believe in yourself. Believe in your solution. Be alert. Keep a positive attitude. Be persistent. Check the feedback. Progress sequentially:

1. How will I develop trust?

2. How will I get my prospect to discover, and verbalize his own needs or wants?

3. What features, and benefits, might I show him that answers, his needs, or wants?

4. How can I help my prospect compare his real alternatives?

5. If my prospect wants to "investigate" thoroughly. . .am I prepared?

6. How can I help my prospect attain confirmation, that my idea is best?

7. What is a good "now incentive"?

8. What is a good close?

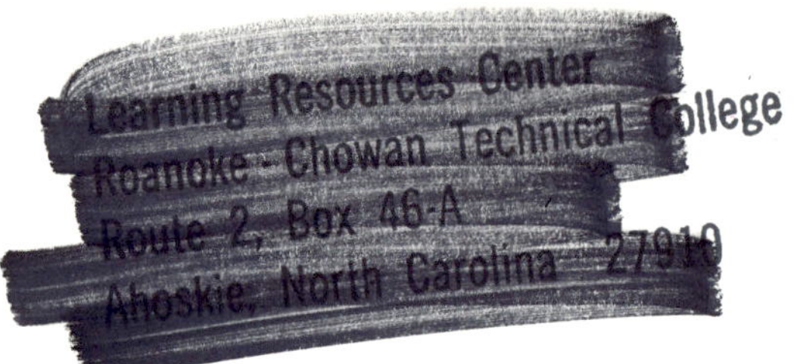